Book Description

How much do you know about exercise, and how to do it in a proper and healthy way?

Exercising can be one of the easiest things to start, but one of the trickiest things to become a master of. You need to have a certain level of understanding of how your body reacts to exercise, as well as having a set of habits in place to continue your journey long-term.

Maybe you have tried picking up an exercise routine in the past, only to struggle to maintain it in the long term, and slowly watch your results drift away. This can be extremely demotivational, and it can make it really hard to try again if this happens!

Or perhaps you have never been into exercising, but you want to give it a try. You are probably aware that people often give up on their exercise plans, so you want to give yourself the best chance to succeed by learning how to workout and how to stick to a plan.

If this sounds like you, then *Change For Good, The Road To Your Own Lifestyle* is the book you won't want to miss out on! It is packed with everything that you need to know about how to get the most out of your exercise, and how to set yourself a plan that you will be able to maintain over time.

Once you begin to understand how to exercise properly and what the potential is for you if you do, you will be amazed at just how much benefit you see from as little as three thirty-minute workouts a week!

The more time you invest into studying the important information covered in this book, the more chance you will give yourself of being able to establish an exercise plan that you can truly stick to, without having to make major changes to your lifestyle.

After all, exercise should fit into your lifestyle, not the other way around!

Inside *Change For Good, The Road To Your Own Lifestyle* discover:

- The importance of push day, and what is involved in that workout day

- The importance of pull day, and what is involved in that workout day

- The importance of leg day, and what is involved in that workout day

- How to work your abdominals and the various benefits that come from strengthening abdominal muscles

- How to make your heart healthier, and the importance of doing so

- How vital your forearm and hand strength is to being able to lift heavy weights and not get injured

- The steps you need to take to not get injured, and how to avoid common exercise mistakes that many people make

- **Why it is important to have a life philosophy, and how to set your own**

And much, much more!

The time has come to stop the endless circle of starting to exercise more frequently, only to give up a month later and end up back at square one.

Instead, invest in yourself and your body and implement a simple workout plan that will change your life for the better.

Don't put off learning this essential information any longer! Grab a copy of *Change For Good, The Road To Your Own Lifestyle* today, and help make your life a better one today.

Change For Good, The Road To Your Own Lifestyle

But First, Exercise

Steve D.

Table of Contents

SKETCH
YOUR LIFESTYLE

YOUR JOURNAL !!!

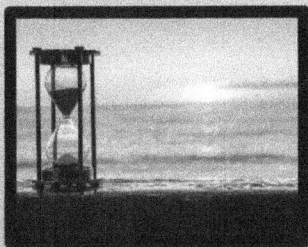

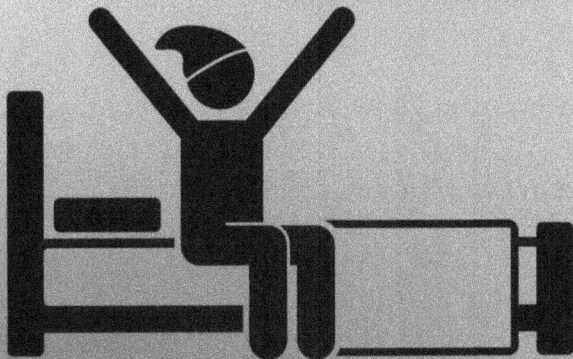

A Special Gift To Our Readers

Included with your purchase of this book is our
Workout Journal Calendar Checklist.

This checklist will help you get started on your
journey.

Click the link below and let us know what email
address to deliver it to.

www.stevedbooks.com

Introduction

*"If you spend too much time thinking about a thing,
you'll never get it done."* - Bruce Lee

Having exercise as part of your weekly, if not daily,
routine is absolutely essential for anyone who is
looking to live a long and healthy life.

It is essential that we bear in mind that we originate
from nomadic ancestors, who used to spend most of
their time moving, often in search of shelter and food.
As a result, they tended to travel large distances each
and every day. Because of this, our bodies are sculpted
and ready to be regularly active.

Similar to a sports car, and the fact that it has been
created to go fast, our bodies have been designed to

move. If you only take a sports car out for a small trip around your town center once every week or so, then it is likely to start showing engine problems pretty fast.

This is no different for people. Over time you are likely to develop issues if you sit down for long periods every day, either in front of your work computer or while watching television, and only exercise a small amount each day.

There are so many different benefits that come from exercising, which is why it is such an important part of anyone's weekly routine. Exercise helps you increase your energy levels, improves your muscle strength, and can help you maintain a healthy weight. Not only that, but it also helps improve your brain function and the health of your heart and body.

With this in mind, I felt it was necessary to offer an insight into how to get a good exercise routine in place, without changing your lifestyle drastically. All too often, diet plans and workout plans are too extreme, asking you to give up major parts of your lifestyle as a sacrifice.

What does this mean? Ultimately this is not a sustainable lifestyle change as you will either quickly become demotivated, or start to associate exercise as a chore, rather than a choice.

I am here to tell you that doesn't have to be the case! There is a way to integrate exercise into your life without the major sacrifices, and build habits that make your plan easy to follow and most importantly, fun!

Before we get into the breakdown of the chapters, I just want to briefly introduce myself. I grew up and still live in New York City and I have a passion for living a healthy lifestyle. In the past, I wasn't very healthy and after a couple of health scares from being very overweight, I decided to make a change. I started eating right and exercising whenever I could. I changed my life for the better and because of this, I'm interested in helping people also change their lives for the better. I want to inspire you to take control of your physical health through exercise, and this book is my way to do that. Now, let's break down what this book will teach you.

Inside chapter one, I will walk you through what a typical "push" day looks like, focusing on your triceps, chest, and shoulder muscles. Inside this chapter, I will start by explaining in more detail what your tricep, chest, and shoulder muscles are, as this will give you a much better grasp on what you are working on and why when you are training. I will also lay out the concept of a push, pull, legs, and rest routine, and how that routine will allow you to gain muscle, without exercise taking over your life.

After we have touched on that concept, we will run through what makes up the push-pull-legs routine, and the benefits of undertaking that exercise program.

If that wasn't enough, I will also explain some of the best exercises you can do to help grow your triceps, whether that is in the gym or at home. The idea of this ebook is that the exercises are accessible for anyone, regardless of whether they are a regular gym goer or not.

I will also explain some of the common mistakes that people make when they are training their triceps, and highlight some of the ways that you can avoid getting injured while training. You may have experienced how frustrating it is to train and then get injured, and how hard it can be to start all over again once the injury has subsided.

We will also touch on exercises you can do at home or in the gym for working your chest muscles, and your shoulder muscles, and the mistakes that people make when training these muscles, and how to avoid injuring them as well.

After we have covered off which muscles you will work during push day, it is time to move onto pull day, which focuses on your back and bicep muscles. In this chapter, I will explain how to get bigger biceps, and the common mistakes people make when they want to grow their biceps but they are struggling to do so. Hint, you need to work all of your bicep from every angle. That means you can't get away with just doing bicep curls!

Here, I will lay out my four rules that you need to follow to help get yourself bigger biceps. Once that is covered, we will move on to the different muscles that make up your back, to give you a great understanding of what you are working on when you are training your back.

I will also touch on why it is called pull day in more detail. The idea is to provide you with as much information as I can so that you don't simply follow what is in this book, you use it to understand working out in greater detail. This greater detail will lead to more motivation when you hit your training sessions.

Now that you have an excellent understanding of how to train your back and biceps, it is time to take you through the different exercises you can do to work your biceps. Rather than in some books, where they simply tell you to do bicep curls, I have laid out a number of different exercises you can do to work your entire bicep, to give you more size and more muscular definition. I have also highlighted some of the common mistakes that people make when they are training their biceps, and how you can avoid them. We will then run through the different exercises you can do to train your back, both in the gym and at home, so there's no excuse not to get your workouts in!

Chapter three is completely dedicated to training your legs. This is the third important aspect of the push, pull, and legs training program. Here, I will go through the different muscles that make up your legs, and which ones are the most important for you to train and get stronger. There are so many different exercises that you can do for leg training, so I have tried to highlight the most beneficial ones that will help you improve your leg strength.

With so much content online these days and easily accessible through social media, it can be all too easy to try out leg workouts that may look cool, but can actually be very damaging to your body, or have minimal impact on your leg strength. Don't believe everything you see on the internet after all!

Therefore, I have also highlighted exercises that you should avoid on leg day, and why they can be more harmful than beneficial.

Next up its abs. Looking for a killer six-pack? This chapter is the one for you! I will take you through the different abdominal muscles, and how each of them makes up your six-pack physique. There is a lot more to getting abs than simply doing crunches!

I will outline some of the main exercises that you can do to work on your abs. You would be amazed at how many different exercises there are that you can do at home or in the gym that work different parts of your abs.

Your core is essential for almost all movements and other strength exercises that you want to tackle, so it's important that you don't skip out on your abdominal workouts! Make sure you also pay attention to the common mistakes that occur when people are training their abs, and how you can avoid these to make sure you are getting the best results possible from your workouts.

Chapter five takes a slightly different turn, focusing on an area that many people overlook in their workout plans, which is your hands. I will take you through the different muscles that make up your hands and wrists, and why it is essential that you strengthen these muscles to allow yourself to lift heavier weights on push, pull, and leg day.

To do this, I will highlight the different exercises that you can do to train your hands and forearms effectively. These exercises can be done in the gym, or even just at home while you wait for the kettle to boil!

I will also outline how to prevent yourself from getting injured while you undergo these exercises. A bad wrist injury could potentially put you out for weeks!

The next muscle that we are going to focus on in this book is the heart. All too often people make mistakes when they are training their heart muscle through cardiovascular training. How often have you started running more times a week, only to quickly lose motivation and give up in a matter of weeks? This can be seriously demotivating and stop you from trying again in the future.

I'm here to tell you that you are not alone. Many of us have gone through the cycle of doing more cardio one week, only to become less active in just a matter of weeks. The good news is that it doesn't have to be this way any longer!

In this chapter, I will take you through the anatomy of your heart, and its important function within your body. There are many conditions that affect your heart, and regular exercise can reduce the chances of getting any of these significantly. In this chapter I will take you through each of the main heart conditions, and how they impact you if you let them. After this, I will also provide you with advice on how to live heart-healthy, which includes adding regular cardio into your week of training.

That doesn't mean going all out on a spin bike in the gym or on a treadmill, it can be as little as going for a walk with your dog or other half! As well as this, I will also highlight some of the common mistakes that people make, and how if you don't do it correctly you could become injured.

After we have gone through all of the different exercises that you can add to your workout regime, it is time to touch on the important topic of stretching. In chapter seven, I will take you through why people should stretch, and the impact that occurs when we do stretch. A lot of people dismiss the importance of stretching when actually it is essential to get the most out of your training, and also to prevent injury.

I will explain to you just how flexible you need to be, and how injuries tend to occur. This section should give you an idea of how to avoid getting injured by stretching more frequently.

So, should you stretch before exercising? I will discuss this topic in great detail so that you have a much better understanding of how important it is to stretch before you train, and the benefits that come from doing so.

It is also important to stretch after you have exercised, so I will make sure that we run through that topic as well in this chapter, as well as looking into the common stretching mistakes that people make, and how to avoid making those mistakes.

Finally, I will discuss why you should set your very own life philosophy. This may be a relatively new concept to you, but by the end of this chapter you should have everything you need to know about setting a life philosophy, and you should be motivated to sit down and make those necessary changes!

Having a life philosophy will give you a focal point for your exercise, which will help keep you motivated while you are training.

So, without further ado, let's dive right in and get started in changing your life for the better, through the great benefits of exercise.

Chapter 1: Push Day: Triceps, Chest, and Shoulders

The Concept of the Push, Pull, Legs and Rest Routine for Muscle Gains

For decades, the push-pull-legs routine has been one of the most used workout splits for gym-goers. Almost all time-provide muscle and strength-building programs fall into this mold, and that isn't likely to change any time soon.

The main reason that push-pull-legs programs have stayed relevant is that they train each major muscle group while also leaving plenty of time for recovery. They can also be tailored to fit your training goal or schedule and are easy to understand.

So if you are seeking to gain strength and muscle as fast as possible, and you don't mind doing some compound lifting, then push-pull-legs is a great workout regime to try.

What Is the Push-Pull-Legs

Routine?

The push-pull-legs routine, also referred to as the PPL split, is a type of weightlifting plan that has you doing three types of workout.

Your push sessions focus on any muscles in your upper body that perform a pushing motion, such as your triceps, shoulders, and pecs.

In a well-planned PPL program, each push workout will focus mainly on dumbbell and barbell bench press, overhead press, dips, and isolated tricep exercises.

Pull workouts focus more on the muscles in your upper body that perform a pulling motion, like your biceps and back muscles. These workouts consist of deadlifts, dumbbells, and barbell rows, pull-ups, pull-downs, and isolated bicep exercises.

Finally, your leg workouts look at working your hamstrings, calves, glutes, and quads.

These workouts focus mainly on squats, lunges, and other isolation exercises. Your core is indirectly worked through your compound lifts, which is why it is not included.

What are the Benefits of Push-Pull-

Legs?

There are many reasons why a PPL routine is commonplace for powerlifters and bodybuilders. As with any good weightlifting plan, PPL has you spending a lot of time on compound exercises.

Compound exercises are exercises that tackle multiple big muscle groups and need you to develop whole-body strength. For example, squatting needs you to use your hamstrings, glutes, quadriceps, and lower back to complete a repetition.

But an exercise such as Russian Leg curls focuses on your glutes and hamstrings, which is why it is not seen as a compound exercise. Compound exercises are essential as they are much better than isolation exercises when it comes to size and strength.

Not only are they more efficient when it comes to how many muscle groups you train per exercise, but they also let your lift heavier loads safely. The only issue with doing more heavy compound lifts is that it asks a lot of your body.

That is why with PPL, you split your upper body training into separate training sessions and keep your lower body training limited each week.

That way, you have plenty of time for your muscles to recover, allowing you to perform to a better standard over time.

Another big plus to PPL is that you customize it to suit your specific training needs. With just three workouts to pick from, it is easy to pick and mix up workouts where needed each week.

One thing to bear in mind, though, is to not attempt this type of routine if you are not eating enough food for your muscles to recover. If you're new to weightlifting, start the routine without weights and focus on the form. You could also have someone watch you to make sure your form is correct before adding light weights.

With all of this in mind, we're going to start with a push day, focusing on the triceps, chest, and shoulders.

What are the Tricep Muscles?

The triceps brachii is one of the main muscles in the upper arm of your body. They run along your humerus, between your elbow and your shoulder. Alongside your biceps, they allow retraction and extension from your forearm. When you contract your triceps, the forearm extends, and your elbow straightens. If your tricep relaxes and you flex your bicep, your forearm will retract, and your elbow will bend.

The triceps are also used to stabilize your shoulder joint. The shoulder has the largest range of motion compared to any other joint in your body, giving you the power to rotate and turn in many directions.

That being said, greater movability does mean that your shoulder can be quite unstable, and your triceps play an essential role in helping stabilize them.

Triceps Location

As I have already touched on, the triceps brachii is a muscle that can be found in your upper arm. If we were to be more specific, it could be found at the back of your upper arm, sitting between your shoulder and your elbow. As the triceps brachii is made up of three heads, it tends to appear shaped like a horseshoe at the back of your arm.

Triceps Function

The primary function of your triceps brachii is to allow your forearm to extend at the elbow. This allows the triceps brachii functions to make your arm straighten at your elbow joint.

What are the Chest Muscles?

Your chest is made up of two large muscles on each side of your chest. These muscles are known as the pectoralis minor and the pectoralis major, and together they are referred to as your pecs.

Here, I will discuss each of these muscles in more detail for your understanding and also cover how you can target each muscle to allow them to get larger and stronger.

Pectoralis Major

When it comes to your two chest muscles, the pectoralis major is the one that covers the majority of your chest. You have one on each side of your chest, each covering half of your upper chest, attaching at your ribs, sternum, humerus, and clavicle.

The pectoralis major is made up of two heads, which both attach to your upper arm. Each head has responsibilities that overlap, as well as distinct functions, which depend on the angle of your upper arm motion.

Sternocostal Head

Starting at the sternum, the sternal head makes up 80 percent of the total size of your major pectoralis.

Because of this, it powers the majority of your muscle actions, rotating your humerus and bringing your arms towards your midline.

Clavicular Head

The upper part of your pectoralis major starts at the clavicle and aids with actions mentioned above, as well as working to flex the humerus.

How to Work the Pec Major

Various exercises can work on a specific head. You can work your sternocostal head using exercises like bench press, dips, and dumbbell flys.

Pectoralis Minor

The pectoralis minor is a smaller, triangular-shaped muscle that is located below the pectoralis major and, even though it sits on your front, it controls structures along with your backside. As well as being attached to your ribs, the pectoralis minor affixes on the coracoid process. The coracoid process is a smaller protrusion that is the shape of a hook and sits on top of your shoulder blade. Because of these attachment points, your pectoralis minor is able to pull down and spread your shoulder blades apart, which aids with breathing.

The pectoralis minor works every time you activate your pectorals, so isolating it can be very tricky.

However, you will be able to focus on your pectoral minor by doing upper body exercises whereby your body is leaned forward and shoulder blades are pulled downward.

To increase growth, you should work your chest twice a week, with at least forty-eight hours for recovery between chest workouts.

What are the Shoulder Muscles?

In total, the shoulder is made up of eight muscles that are attached to the humerus, scapula, and clavicle. They mold the outer shape of your underarm and shoulder. The muscles that make up your shoulder support in a range of movement and also protect and maintain your main shoulder joint.

The biggest shoulder muscle is the deltoid. This huge triangular muscle is what gives your shoulder the rounded-off shape. It stretches over the top of your shoulder, from the scapular at the back to the clavicle at the front.

From there, it stretches down to the center of your humerus bone. A range of fibers from the muscle is in charge of many different actions, such as raising your arm. One of the main functions of your deltoid is stopping you from dislocating your joint if you carry something heavy.

Different Exercises for the Triceps

In the Gym

Close-grip Bench Press

This type of bench press is an excellent tricep exercise. While a normal bench press works your core and chest, putting your hands closer to each other brings the triceps into play, making them work harder, which leads to more tricep strength and growth.

How to do it:
Grab a barbell using an overhand grip, with your hands shoulder-width apart. Hold the bar over your sternum, with your arms completely straight.

Then, lower your bar straight down towards your head, pause for a second, and then push the bar back towards its starting position.

Rope Tricep Pushdown

The rope tricep pushdown, when done correctly, hones in on your triceps. If you take on too much weight, then you will engage your shoulder and back muscles, which is not what we are trying to achieve here.

How to do it:

Attach a rope handle onto the cable station high pulley. Bend your arms and pick up the rope with an overhand grip. Your hands should be shoulder-width apart. Keep your upper arms tucked into your sides.

Keeping your upper arms fixed, push the rope down until you have locked out elbows. Return to the start position slowly.

Tricep Dips (Advanced)

As you are lifting your total body weight, your triceps are forced to work against a heavier load than they normally would have to with a tricep-isolation exercise.

How to do it:

Lift yourself up onto parallel bars, making sure your torso is perpendicular to the floor.

Cross your ankles and bend your knees before lowering your body slowly until your shoulder joints are lower than your elbows.

Then, push up until your elbows are close to locking out at the top.

Overhead Triceps Extension

As you work on your triceps, it may slip your mind that there are three aspects to the muscle: the medial head, the lateral head, and the long head. The long head doesn't always get enough attention unless you do overhead tricep extensions often.

How to do it:

Pick up a dumbbell and sit on a bench. Create a diamond shape with each hand to grip the top of the dumbbell. Raise it above your head before lowering the dumbbell down by bending at your elbow, keeping your shoulders static. Raise the weight all the way up to overhead by extending your arms.

Skullcrushers (Lying Triceps Extensions)

While there are plenty of ways to make this move, an elbow extension is important in each and every rep. As your upper arms become locked, the lateral and long tricep heads are being used.

How to do it:
Grab an EZ bar by the inner grips, with an overhand grip. Extend your arms up, filling over your chest while lying on a bench. Without moving your elbows, lower the bar towards your forehead. Push back to the starting position to complete a repetition.

At Home

The Diamond Push-up

There are not many more basic tricep exercises than this one. A normal push-up works your chest and arms, but if you bring your hands closer together, the focus shifts to your triceps.

How to do it:
Bring yourself down into a normal push-up starting position before bringing your hands together under your chest, thumbs and forefingers touching each

other. Lower towards the ground, then push back up to the original position.

Bench Dip (Basic)

If you aren't able to do conventional dips, you could try to out bench dips. Ensure you go down slowly, creating more time under tension, then explode back up.

How to do it:
Stand with the bench behind you, grabbing it with each hand placed shoulder-width apart. Extend your legs straight out in front of you. Lower your body by bending at your elbows until your forearm and arm make a 90-degree angle. Push back up to the starting position with your triceps.

Dumbbell Floor Press

This type of bench press is beneficial for the lockout aspect of the lift, which engages your triceps a lot. Since the load sits differently than if it was a barbell, your stabilizing muscles are required to work harder to maintain the position of the weight.

How to do it:

Get a dumbbell in each hand and lay flat on the ground. Hold your dumbbells above your head, and then bend your arms to lower the dumbbells.

Once your elbows have gently touched the ground, press the weights back up.

The Classic Push-up

Sometimes the old exercises and the best ones. A traditional push-up works your core, your chest, and your triceps. The benefit of a push-up is that it can be done anywhere.

How to do it:

Get into the push-up position with your weight on your toes and your hands directly below your shoulders, keeping your body straight. Make sure you keep your core engaged and your body in a straight line.

Lower your chest towards the floor, and then drive your chest back up until you are back in the starting position.

One Arm Kettlebell Floor Press

By only working one arm at a time, we will isolate your triceps, so they are forced to work hard.

How to do it:
Lie down on the floor, holding a kettlebell in one hand, and your upper arm fully extended above your head towards the ceiling.

Bring your arm down to the floor as you would a dumbbell press before pushing the kettlebell up to the ceiling to complete the rep.

Common Mistakes and how to Avoid Injury

Failure to Add in Close-Grip Bench Presses and Dips

Don't get me wrong, isolation exercises definitely have a role to play in tricep programs, but you won't ever reach your full potential without also adding dips and close-grip bench presses to your program.

Failure to Include Overhead Movements

The long head of your tricep is the majority of its mass, and this part activates the best exercises in which your arms are overhead, and your elbows are up near your ears. Each tricep workout should therefore have some form of overhead exercise included, such as cable extensions or overhead barbell.

Using the Same Volume for Tris as Bis

Don't get me wrong, I'm fully aware that a lot of people prefer to train biceps than triceps, but as triceps are more complex muscles, they do need to be worked more to reach their full development. I would always suggest you work the same volume for bis and tris, if not even more tris.

Wild Elbows

If you are looking to grow muscle as quickly as possible, then you need to ensure your muscle is getting the most tension from each rep. A lot of people tend to let their elbows move during extensions or pushdowns, which utilizes other muscle groups. Make sure you keep them tight at all times.

Not Locking Out

The majority of triceps muscle fiber firing takes place in the final third of the press, extension, or pushdown. Therefore, if you don't lock your arms out, you will not be engaging your triceps fully and could be missing out on hypertrophy. Ensure that you lock out while under full control to utilize and work your triceps fully.

Different Exercises for the Chest

In the Gym

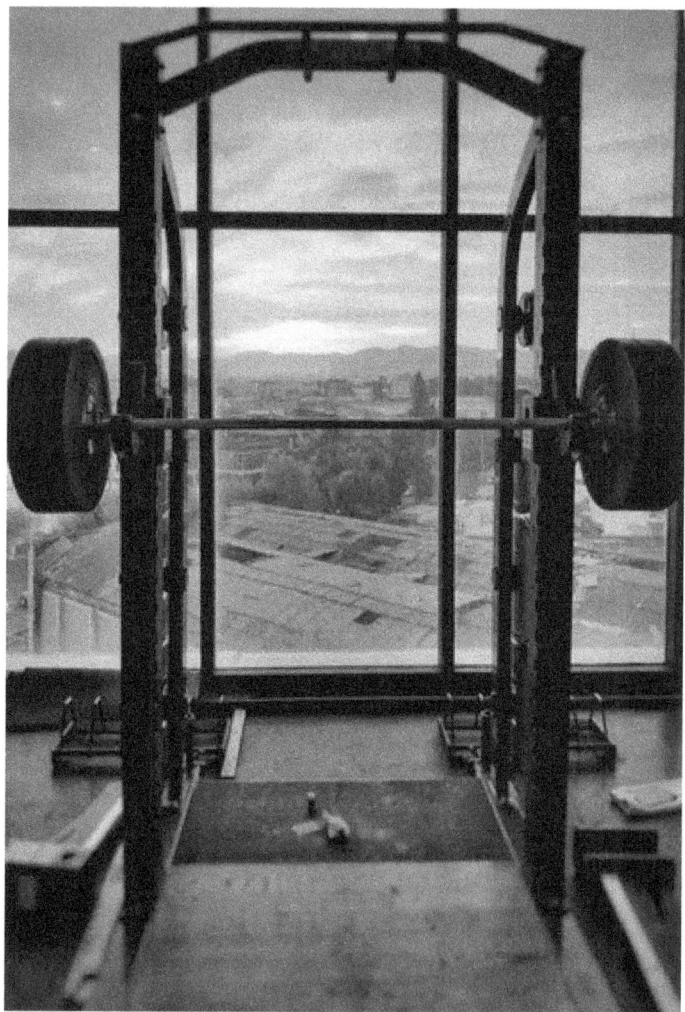

Barbell Bench Press

The most power can be generated from barbell lifts, so the simple barbell bench press allows you to lift the most weight. It is also a simple lift to control, rather than using heavy dumbbells. It is easy to learn, and you can have a spotter for when it gets heavy.

You should do it towards the beginning of your workout for heavy sets and minimal reps. Think about varying your grip for full chest development.

Flat Bench Dumbbell Press

Bench pressing with dumbbells means that each side of your body is forced to work independently, which makes your stabilizing muscles work harder, as dumbbells are hard to control.

Dumbbells allow a longer range of motion than you can get with a barbell. By doing it on a flat bench, you can lift heavy weights and make a nice alternative to a barbell bench.

Incline Barbell Bench Press

Often you will notice that benches tend to be fixed at a particularly steep angle, which needs a larger contribution from your delts rather than your chest. Where you can, choose a less-steep incline to make sure you are hitting your upper pectorals. A smith machine is excellent for this type of movement.

If you're focusing on building up your upper chest, you can bring your grip closer to attack those upper-chest fibers more.

Almost all chest workouts begin with a flat bench and then move on to an incline bench, but it's time to change that. Mix things up and start with inclines; you'll lift more as you feel fresher and put more focus on your upper pectoralis fibers.

Machine Decline Press

Some machines that you can find in the gym, such as the hammer strength, lets you move each of your arms on their own, which is excellent for a chest day workout. As well as performing a machine decline press from straight on, you could also sit sideways on the machine, pressing across the body.

Seated Machine Chest Press

While I would always recommend making some free-weight pressing moves from a flat bench, there are some unique benefits to machine presses as well. For starters, they are excellent for controlling your reps and also make a great tool for completing drop sets.

I would add machine exercises to the back end of any workout, as they provide you with more chance of pumping your pectoralis without any shoulder assistance.

At Home

Regular Push-ups

This classic exercise is a great home workout to start with and should be in any upper-body workout. Ensure you use a wide grip, as this works your chest muscles more than other techniques.

Incline Push-ups

If you struggle with a normal push-up, then you could try incline push-ups. The more the incline, the easier the exercise is to complete. Try this out to build yourself up to regular push-up.

Decline Push-ups

Decline push-ups allow you to specifically target your deltoid and upper chest muscles. They also put more of your body weight into the exercise, compared to a normal push up, which makes them more difficult.

Plyometric Push-ups

Are you keen to explode into action? Plyometric push-ups can be done in several great ways, such as clap push-ups. These short sharp bursts of plyometric movement will make your muscles fire on all cylinders.

Time Under Tension Push-ups

You may not believe this, but by slowing down a movement or paying more attention to form, you will get much greater results. Dropping yourself slowly into a push-up and then rising slowly will help you gain muscle mass.

Common Mistakes and how to Avoid Injury

Elbows Too High

As you bench press with each elbow out directly sideways, you are putting great strain on your elbows and shoulder. This also means the barbell will come to your collarbones rather than your chest, making the movement much tougher as a result.

Grip the bar narrower and keep your elbows in tighter to your rib cage, at about 45 degrees rather than 90 degrees.

Bouncing the Bar

At the bottom part of any bench press, make sure that you aren't bouncing the bar off your body; this gives you extra momentum and makes the bar easier to lift, but you could damage your rib cage if the weight is heavy.

If you need to bounce your barbell, then it is probably too heavy. Lower the weight and don't bounce for maximum strength gains.

Not Squeezing Your Shoulders

The bench press requires more than simply lying down and pushing the weight. You need to ensure you have a stable foundation to lift from and make it as efficient as you can.

If you don't slide your shoulder blades together, then you will be reducing your chest activation, making the shoulders work harder. Always make sure your shoulder blades are locked back and down when pressing.

Not Getting a Liftoff

Without getting liftoff, it can be tricky to bring your barbell to the starting position while keeping your posture. For example, when you lift the weight out of the rack, your shoulders have to round, and you will lose your upper back tension. Once the bar is over your body, it's impossible to pull your blades back together.

Instead, get into the correct position, and ask a partner to hand you the barbell. If you don't have a spotter, try and put a rack there so you aren't forced to lose your posture.

Not Pausing Before Descent

Once you have started and you have the bar held at the top, try and avoid the urge to instantly start your bench press. Pause for a second, that way, you will sink and lock your body, which creates more stability for your press. It will also up the tension in your body for more gains.

Not Using Your Legs

When you bench press, make sure you don't flail your legs or tap your feet. Instead, dig your feet into the ground as you set up and set a firm foundation. Make sure you also squeeze your glutes and tense your quads to help lift more weight.

Breaking Your Wrists

How you grip the barbell will be the maker or breaker of your lift. Make sure you don't grip it too high up in your palm or just in your fingertips. If you do, you will lose strength, and you will injure your wrists as the barbell strains your joints and tendons.

Make sure the barbell is set deep into your palm, with your wrists ever so slightly bent.

Lifting Your Hips off the Bench

By lifting your hips off the bench, you create an arch in your body from your feet all the way to your shoulder, which puts a big strain on your spine. Make sure you keep your glutes in contact with the bench instead of arching your upper back. This is a safer and better lifting position.

Lifting Your Head off the Bench

Make sure your head is on the bench at all times when performing a bench press. By lifting up, you are putting a strain on your neck, as well as wasting energy. If you find it hard to keep your neck down, then you may have a forward-neck posture. If this is the case, hold off on training your chest until you have alleviated the imbalances that make your neck come forwards.

Shortening Your Range-of-Motion

If you choose to only lower the barbell a little bit, you will miss out on strength and muscle gains. Less range of movement will not have the same results, even if you are lifting heavier weights. Ensure each rep touches your chest.

Different Exercises for the Shoulders

In the Gym

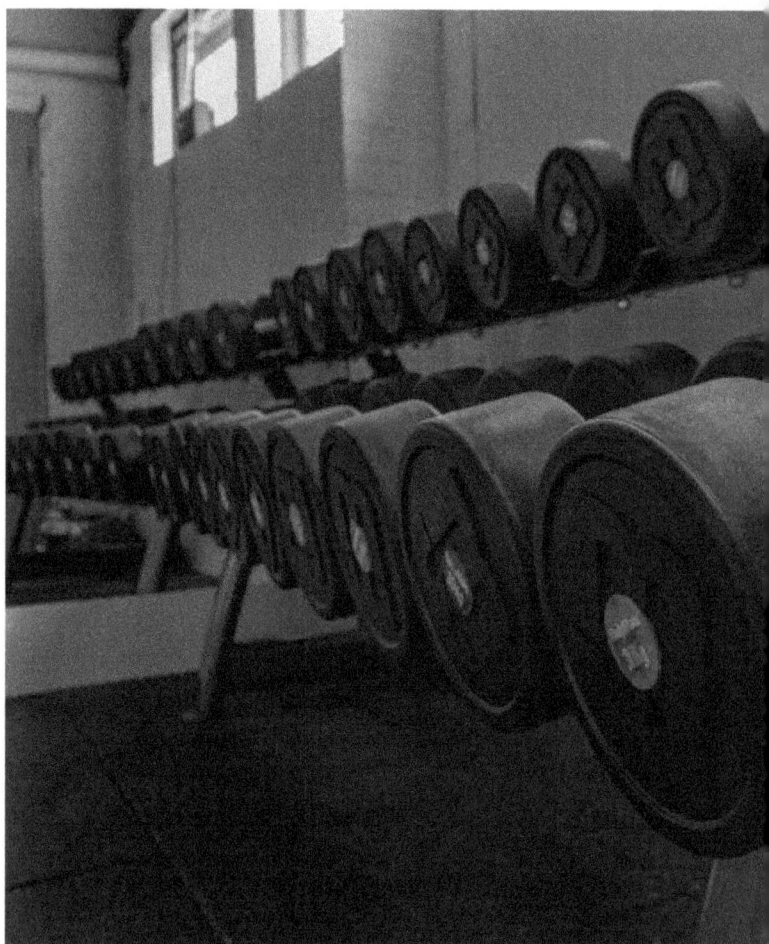

Seated Overhead Dumbbell Press

This exercise lets you utilize each of the three shoulder muscles in one. An added bonus is that this movement also works your triceps. In the seated position, pick up two dumbbells and lift them to your ears, with your elbows at a 90-degree bend, before pushing up.

Ensure that your elbows aren't fully locked out at the top of each rep, as it can cause injury to your joints.

Plate Press out

Plate press outs don't require a barbell; all you need is a heavily weighted plate that will challenge you. Hold the plate at around nine and three o'clock, and keep it close to your chest. Extend your arms in front of you, and then bring them back to your chest.

Lateral Raises

When completing a lateral raise, you don't need lots of weight, so this isn't an exercise for any ego-lifters out there! Start by standing and holding a workable weight in both hands, down to your sides. Raise both hands up and away from you to the point that your arms are parallel to the ground. Lower slowly to the start position to finish the rep.

Shoulder Shrugs

Shoulder shrugs are a simple yet effective movement for you to take advantage of. Grab a weight in each hand before shrugging your shoulders up and down with control. The weight should be testing, but it should also be achievable to do at least 12 repetitions per set.

At Home

Diving Dolphin

The diving dolphin lets you engage your anterior deltoids without the need for any equipment. It is also excellent for improving your shoulder stability, as it utilizes your shoulders through a closed-chain movement. This is because your hands and feet are fixed during the exercise.

Begin in the forearm plank, with your elbows below your shoulders and no wider than your hips. Bring your feet towards your arms so that your hips move towards the ceiling.

Bring your hips down and keep your body in a flat line, driving your shoulders forward so that you hover over your wrists.

Plank Raise Crunches

If you are looking for another closed-chain exercise that is good for shoulder stability is plank raise crunches. As well as working your shoulders, this exercise is also excellent for your core.

Begin in straight arm plank position, shoulders above your palms, and your feet shoulder-width apart. Bring your right arm forward, and then bring it back down. Bring your right arm to the side, then bring it back down.

Maintain a straight line with your body as you bring your left arm below your body and pull your right leg up to your core, touching your hand and foot. Return to the original position for a full rep.

Dumbbell Lateral Raise

This exercise is great for targeting your middle deltoid. Stand upright with your feet shoulder-width apart, keeping your arms to your sides, with a dumbbell in each hand.

Bring your arms to your sides until they are level with the shoulder, with your palms pointing downwards.

Lower your arms slowly before repeating.

Reverse Fly

While this is mainly an upper back exercise, it can also be used to engage your posterior deltoid. Stand with your feet under your shoulders, gripping a dumbbell in each of your hands.

Bend forward over your hips, to the point that your chest is almost parallel to the ground. Let the weights hang down to the ground, palms facing inwards. From there, keep your back flat and raise your arms out to each side until they are as high as your body.

Military Press

The military press focuses on your entire deltoid muscle and is great for muscle growth. It also works your trap, triceps, and pectoral muscles. Stand upright with your feet hip-width apart and a dumbbell in both of your hands. Step forward slightly with one foot.

Bring the weights to shoulder height, palms facing forwards.

Extend your arms up and over your head, keeping your back straight and engaging your core. Lower the weights to shoulder height to complete the repetition.

Chapter 2: Pull Day: Biceps and Back

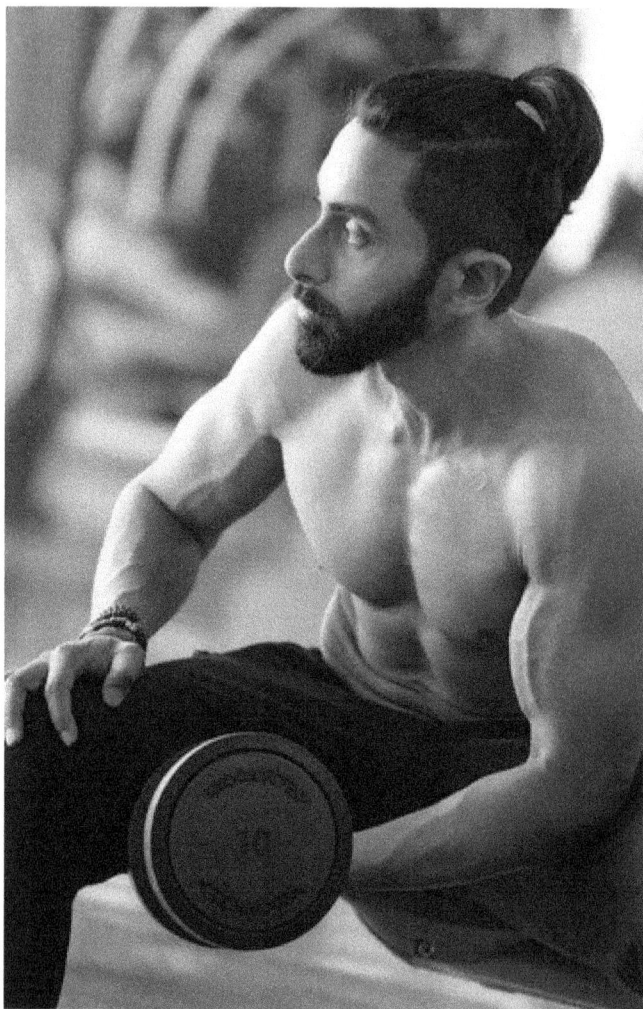

Why is it Called Pull Day?

Pull workout exercises are strength movements that create a concentric contraction. This is where the muscles are shorted while you move two connection points nearer to each other. For example, hamstring curls, pull-ups, or bicep curls.

Pull exercises are the complete opposite of push ones, which are exercises that lengthen your muscle. While there are several exercises that are depicted as pull or push exercises, in truth, almost all exercises have a concentric and an eccentric phase. For example, when you complete a bicep curl, the lifting part is the shortening, and the lowering part is the lengthening.

In the series of push-pull-leg, the pull day includes working with biceps and back.

How to Get Bigger Biceps: Attack From All Angles

We are all seeking bigger biceps. Well, a lot of us anyway! If you are looking to gain bigger biceps, then these exercises will support your gains. If you do them correctly, then you will start to see results before you know it.

Building bigger biceps doesn't have to be tricky. If you are training them often and not seeing results at the moment, then you are likely training them incorrectly, and bicep curls will only take you so far. You may be fascinated to know just how many different training exercises there are out there to work your biceps.

One of the most common reasons that people's biceps do not grow as quickly as they would like them to is because they are unable to realize that the bicep is made up of three different parts: The bicep brachii, which makes up the largest bump in your arm, the brachialis, which is the muscle that sits below the bicep, and the brachioradialis, which is the muscle that runs down the forearm.

A lot of people focus entirely on the brachii. However, if you are looking for fuller, thicker arms, then you need to work on each aspect of the bicep.

Four Rules For Bigger Biceps

Make a note of these important tips to make sure that you are getting the most out of each and every rep. If you are going to spend time working on your biceps, then it is important that you do them properly.

Rule 1: Warm-Up

It may seem rather tedious, but it is essential that you warm up before any lifting, and that is no different for biceps. Simply put, warming up your muscles will make them work better. The increase in the temperature of your bicep will lower the chances of any rips or tears, and you'll be ready to lift more.

Rule 2: Change Up Your Workouts

Remember, once you have done a workout about six times, your body has become adapted to it, and you will stop getting the benefits. Variety keeps your training interesting, and it keeps your muscles on their toes.

Rule 3: The Importance of Breathing

Do you ever hold your breath when you are committing to a big lift? You shouldn't! Structured and controlled breathing allows you to keep calm, concentrate, and keep your tempo under control.

It is also essential that you breathe properly and engage your diaphragm, as it is essential for explosive performance.

Rule 4: Rest More

You may have heard people suggest before that you should try and rest for 30 to 60 seconds after each set. However, this isn't long enough for you to be able to fully recover your muscles. Ideally, you should wait anywhere between three or four minutes, especially when you are lifting heavy.

Back Muscles

The muscles of your back can be split into three groups; deep, superficial, and intermediate. The superficial allows movements of the shoulder, the intermediate allows movements of the thoracic cage, and the deep allows movements of the vertebral column.

The deep muscles are developed embryologically in your back and are known as intrinsic muscles. The intermediate and superficial muscles do not develop in your back and are referred to as extrinsic muscles.

The superficial back muscles can be found under the skin and the superficial fascia. They come from the vertebral column and attach to your shoulder bones. All of these muscles are associated with moving your upper limb.

The muscles in this group are known as the latissimus dorsi, trapezius, rhomboids, and levator scapulae.

Trapezius

A flat, broad, and triangular muscle, the trapezius is the most superficial out of all of the back muscles. The fibers from the upper end of the trapezius lift the scapula before rotating it through the abduction of your arm. The middle fibers allow the scapula to retract, and the scapula is pulled by the lower fibers.

Latissimus Dorsi

The latissimus dorsi starts in the lower part of your back and covers a vast area. The latissimus dorsi is responsible for moving the upper limb. It extends, medially rotates, and adducts.

Levator Scapulae

A small strap-like muscle, the levator scapulae starts at your neck and goes down to attach to your scapular. It is responsible for elevating your scapula.

Rhomboids

In total, there are two rhomboid muscles, the major and the minor. Your Rhomboid major is attached to the medial border of your scapula, in between the inferior angle and the scapula spine. It is used to retract and rotate your scapula. Your rhomboid minor is attached at the media border of your scapula, at the level of the spine. It is used to retract and rotate your scapula.

Exercises for the Biceps

In the Gym

Standing Dumbbell Curl

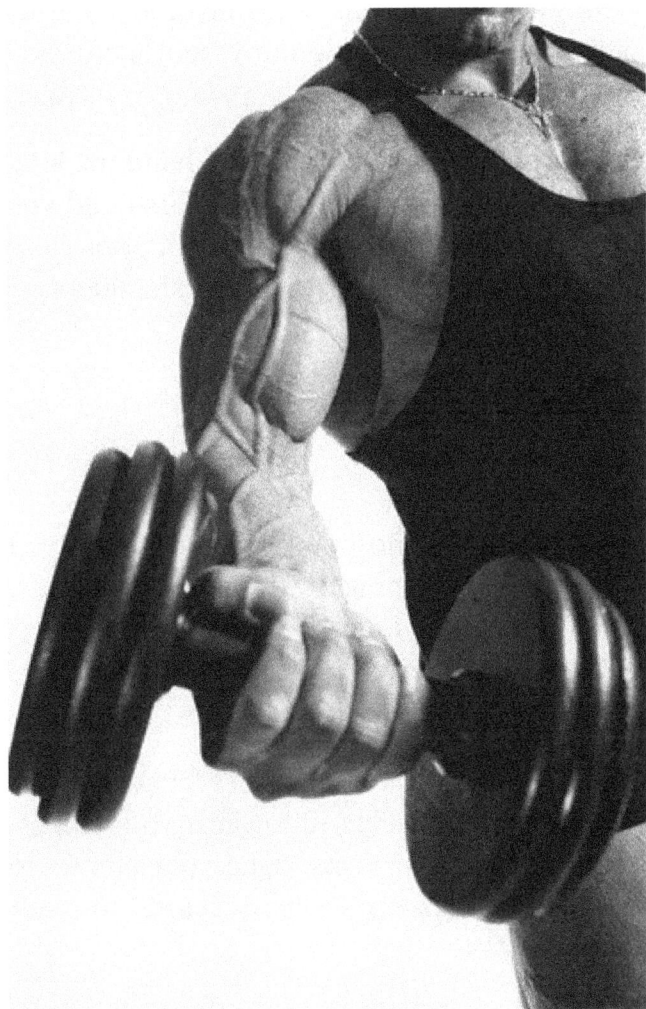

When it comes to bicep exercises, this is the most common and easy to execute to use the standing dumbbell curl. No exercise targets your biceps as much as the dumbbell curl. But you need to make sure that you pick the correct weight to lift.

If you wildly swing your arms and arch your back to lift a dumbbell, then you are wasting your time and may cause yourself injury. Keep the movement controlled and slow.

Stand with a dumbbell hanging in each hand, making sure that your elbows are next to your torso and you have your palms facing forwards. Keep your arms close to your side, and curl the weights to your shoulders.

Hammer Curl

The key here is in detail, most importantly, the way you grip the dumbbell. By turning the dumbbell on its side, it allows you to transfer more focus from your biceps brachii to the brachialis, which is the muscle that gives your arm thickness.

Allow a pair of dumbbells to sit at arm's length by your sides, with your palms facing in towards your thighs. Rather than moving your arms, bend your elbows to curl the dumbbells, keep them as close to your shoulders as you can.

Incline Dumbbell Curl

Place your bench in the incline position, which places added pressure on the long head of your biceps brachii as you are working at a deficit. Simply put, you're beginning at a point where you don't have as much leverage as usual.

Begin by lying with your back on a bench that is laid at a 45-degree angle. Bend your elbows to curl the dumbbells, keeping them as close to your shoulders as possible. Then, lower your dumbbells slowly to the starting place, straightening your arms.

Zottman Curl

There are very few exercises that focus on the three main muscles that make up your bicep. By switching from an underhand to an overhand grip at the halfway point, the zottman curl strikes all areas of the bicep.

With dumbbells by each side, twist your arms, so your palms are facing forwards. Making sure not to move the upper arms, bend the elbows to curl the dumbbell to your shoulder. On the way down, rotate the dumbbell so that your palms are facing forwards.

Decline Dumbbell Curl

By lying on your chest, you will be able to isolate your biceps better, as there is no weight coming through your core or legs. Mix up your grip so that you can target different areas of the bicep.

Lie with your chest down on a bench that is propped at a 45-degree incline. Bend your elbows without moving your upper arms, curling the dumbbells to the shoulder.

Barbell Bent-over Row

It is well-researched that your biceps are at their most active when they are pulling. As a bent-over row needs a lot of muscles to perform, then you are able to pull more weight than you would be able to curl while keeping good form.

With flexed knees, hinge over from your hips, keeping a neutral spine, and have your hands shoulder-width apart. When pulling, try pinching your elbows behind your back.

Chin-up

Not a move that is easy for beginners, but one that is highly effective. When done properly, your arms and shoulders will experience a serious workout.

Grab the rig with your hands facing towards you, with a grip slightly more narrow than your shoulder width. Pull yours up, all the way until your head is over the bar.

Regular EZ Bar Curl

The EZ bar lets you load more weight onto the bar than you would be able to for a normal curl while keeping good form and not putting a lot of pressure through your forearms and elbows.

Keep the EZ bar held in front of your thighs with an underhand grip, shoulder-width apart. When you breathe in, curl the bar up to your shoulders.

Underhand Seated Row

By rowing from a seated position, your biceps are in the perfect position for the pull, making them work even harder with each rep. Perform it properly, and your back and biceps are sure to grow.

Flex your knees and keep the bar held in an underhand grip, with your hands shoulder-width apart. Lean back ever so slightly, making sure your back is straight, before using your back muscles to pull the bar towards your stomach.

Reverse Curl Straight Bar

Reverse curl straight bar is often overlooked as it works the brachialis, a muscle that cannot be seen in your upper arm, but one that is vital if you are looking to grow your biceps. Train it efficiently, and the brachialis will push the peak of your bicep muscle up, giving you a bigger flex and larger arms.

At Home

Grocery Bag Curl

To complete this exercise, you need to have a grocery bag, or perhaps a backpack, and fill it with heavy objects such as books or canned goods.

Hold the handle of your bag by your side, and bend your elbow to bring your back up to your shoulder before lowering it back down. Keep control and ensure your arms don't begin to swing.

Broomstick Curl

Another option is a broomstick curl, whereby your hang weighted bags off each side of the broomstick. Hold it with each hand and curl the broomstick, bending the elbows to take the broomstick up to your shoulder and then back down.

Inverted Row

This one is slightly more tricky. You will need to have access to a sturdy broomstick, along with a couple of sturdy chairs. Lay the broomstick across the two chairs, with room in between them so that you can lie down under the broomstick.

Lie in between the chairs under the broomstick, and use it to pull your body up, keeping only your heels on the floor.

Banded Curl

Lay a resistance band on the floor before standing on it, with your fit hip-width apart. Grab one end of the band in both of your hands, with your hands pointing upwards. Bend at your elbows, lifting the band to your shoulders and then back down, keeping control through the movement.

Banded Hammer Curl

Start positioning your resistance band to perform a standard curl; position your hands so that your palms face each other and your thumbs are facing upwards. Keep your elbows close to your body when you curl.

Banded Reverse Curl

Layout your resistance band as if you were about to do a standard curl, but instead, position your hands so that your palms are facing downwards. Keep your elbows in tight to your body as you curl.

Barbell Biceps Curl

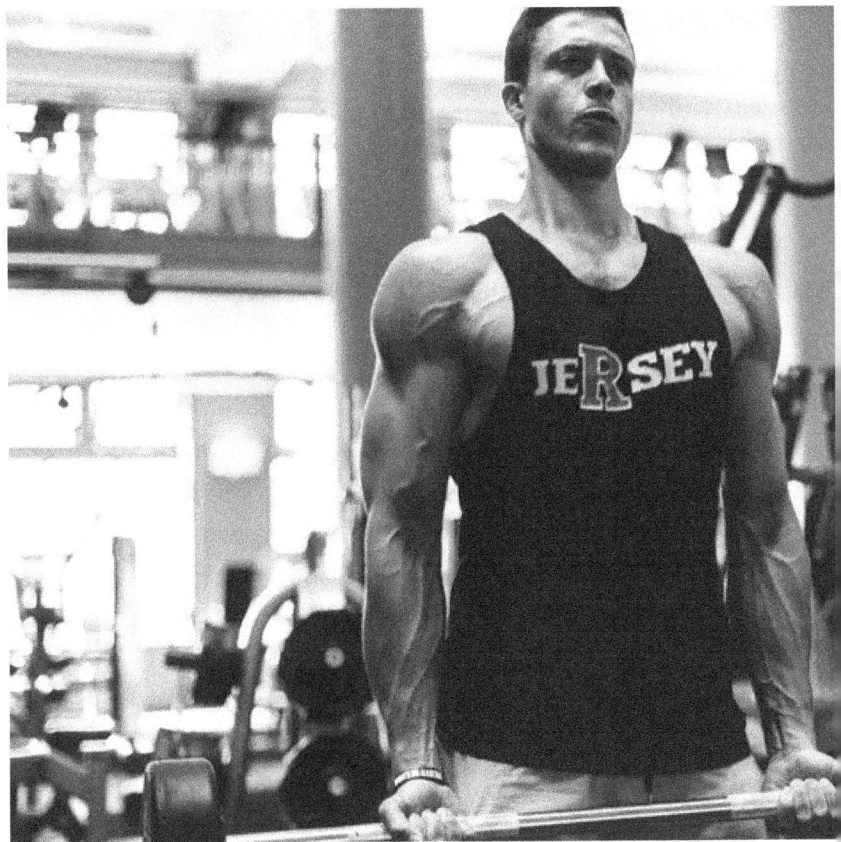

Grip your broomstick with two weighted bags. Slowly bring your hands upward, bending your elbows to do so in a controlled manner.

Reverse-grip Barbell Curl

Set yourself up to complete a standard barbell curl, but instead, grip the broomstick with your hands facing towards the ground. Keep control whilst you curl and lower the broomstick, trying not to swing it.

Supinated-grip Barbell Row

Standing with your knees slightly bent and your feet shoulder-width apart, bend yourself forward up until your spine is at a 45-degree angle to the floor. Grip the broomstick with both hands and straight arms. Pull the elbows back and bring the barbell close to your stomach.

Neutral-grip Pull-up

You will need to have a pull bar for this movement or a set of monkey bars if you can get to a playground. Execute a pull-up with your hands facing inwards towards each other. If you struggle to do a full pull-up, then you can try using a chair as assistance.

Common Mistakes

Too Much Swinging

You have probably seen a few bicep curl swingers in your time at the gym. These are the people who put far too much weight on the bar and then swing around like a see-saw!

Don't get lured in by the big weights.

The activation of your muscle is dependent on the rate of lifting and lowering the weights. Drop your ego and pick a weight that you can manage. You need to be able to contract your biceps at the top of each rep without any swinging.

Using Only One Grip Width

Another mistake often made with barbell exercises is that you only use one grip all the time. Changing how wide your grip does not only add variety to your training but also utilizes other muscles in different ways for further growth and strength.

Mixing up the width of your grip changes the degree of rotation in your upper arm. The wider the grip, the more your arms turn out at the joint. This rotation leads to more focus on inner muscles.

Executing a close grip means that your arms turn in. This rotation activates your outer muscles.

Avoiding Pull-Ups And Chin-Ups

Training your biceps needs more than just barbell curls and dumbbells, although these are very beneficial bicep exercises. Some bodyweight exercises such as pull-ups or chin-ups are known as the foundation of creating bulging biceps. Chin-ups help you create a base of mass and strength in your arms. So switch up your usual pattern of simply doing bicep curls, and look to add in pull-ups and chin-ups into your workout plan.

Letting The Elbows Flare Out

When completing a bicep exercise, make sure you keep an eye on the position of your elbows. A lot of people tend to focus more on their upper arms, forgetting that they need their elbows to stay tight while you are working.

If your biceps move then, you won't get the same work going through your biceps, and it will defeat the purpose of training biceps.

Training Too Frequently

Over-training any muscle group is a mistake, including overtraining your biceps. Biceps are often used on other strength training days, even if they are not targeted specifically. If you train often, then working your biceps three or more times a week will be overkill.

Make sure that you are allowing your biceps time to rest and recover. Not intaking enough protein is also a big mistake. Post-workout shakes using whey powders can offer you everything you need to recover and repair your muscles.

Exercises for Your Back

In the Gym

Barbell Deadlift

Technically, a barbell deadlift is more than just a back exercise, as it engages your full posterior chain, from your calves all the way to your upper traps. But it is a great exercise for backside development. When you deadlift, the technique is absolutely essential and will allow you to lift large weights in no time.

There are several deadlift progression programs that you can follow to gain new personal bests. Stick to a normal barbell deadlift on back day, but you can also use other styles of the deadlift, such as sumo-style, to keep mixing up your workouts.

If you are going to do heavy reps, then make sure you deadlift when you are fresh.

Bent-Over Barbell Row

When it comes to back movements, this one is up there with the best of them, given the sheer amount of weight that you are able to lift. As with the deadlift, this move is another that needs you to have top quality form but rewards you with lots of muscle gains.

You should implement bent-over rows at the beginning of your back workouts for heavy sets and low reps.

Compared to other back exercises, the bent-over barbell row has a more significant lumber load, which is why it is important to do it at the start of your workout.

Wide-Grip Pull-Up

It's always good to have an overhead pulling movement in your back program and pull-ups are one of the very best. Wide-grip pull-ups offer you a great option for emphasizing your upper body. With a close grip, you get a longer range of motion, but you will be able to load your wide-grip pull-ups more as the starting joint position is optimized.

If you add pull-ups to the start of your workout, you could even add a weighted belt. However, if you find them tough, then you can always try using an assisted pull-up machine or switch to wide-grip pull-downs.

Good form is essential here, making sure your scapular is retracted, and you pull your shoulder blades down.

As the pill up a range of motion is a long one, a couple of light reps make for a great warm-up of your shoulder joints.

Standing T-Bar Row

I chose to add the T-bar row rather than a chest-supported version, as it allows you to stack on more weight, even if that tends to cause a little bit of cheating through the hips and knees. For some, it can be tough to try and maintain a flat back; If that is the case for you, then a supported version is a better option.

This is not a squat movement, so make sure that you maintain locked legs in a bend angle. You also need to choose between wide and close grip. A wider grip will allow more emphasis on your lats, and a neutral grip will target your middle back better.

Make sure this workout is done early on in your workout, and focus mainly on the stretch and contraction of your back.

Wide-Grip Seated Cable Row

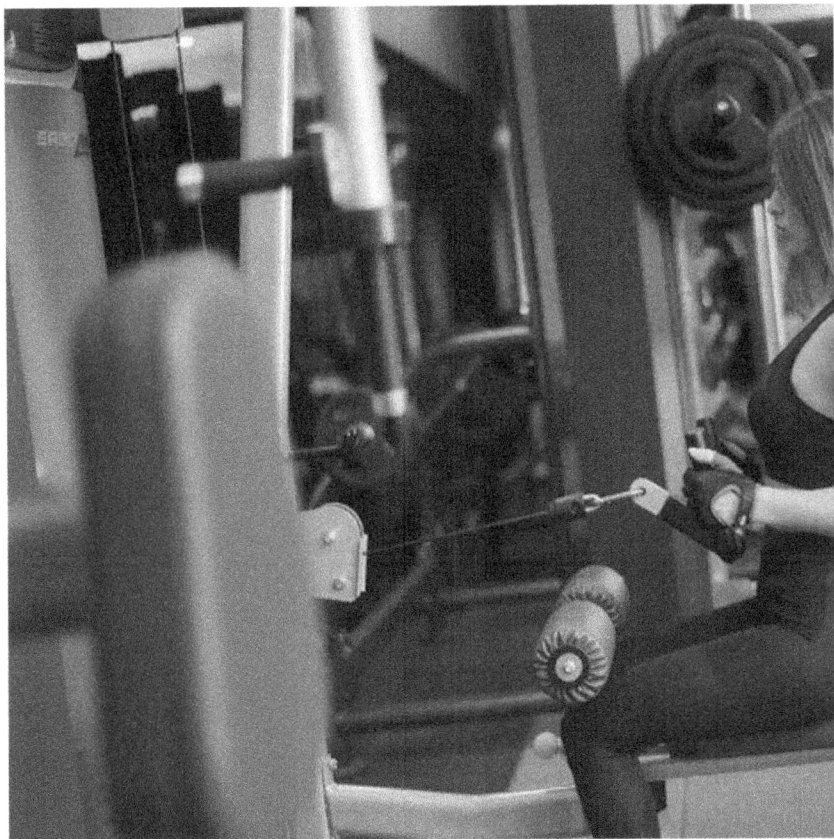

Almost everyone's go-to is a close-grip bar when it comes to rows. If this is something that you do, you will notice that using a wide grip when on a lat bar will make a nice change of pace, as it moves more emphasis onto your upper lats. Wide rows emulate the benefits from some back machines, so be sure not to do both in your workout unless you create some type of variance, such as your grip.

You could even try and reverse your grip, looking at something near shoulder-width apart, which further targets your lower lats, as your elbows stay tucked in at the sides.

At Home

Single-Arm Suitcase Deadlift

Standing with your feet shoulder-width apart, and with a heavy dumbbell placed on the floor next to your right foot, bend down and pick up the dumbbell. The focus here is to drive your body weight through your heels, ensuring that your torso is finished in an upright position. Slowly take the weight back to the ground before repeating.

Dumbbell Swing

Stand with your feet shoulder-width apart, holding a heavy dumbbell in both hands, grabbing it from the top. Move your hips back and bend your knees slightly before lowering your chest and bringing the dumbbell through your legs. Bring your hips forward, swinging the dumbbell up to shoulder height.

Dumbbell Plank Lateral Drag

Lay a dumbbell on the left-hand side of your body. Begin at the top of a press-up position, with your palms on the ground, underneath your shoulders, before walking your feet back all the way until your body is in a straight line from your heels to your shoulders. With your right hand, reach under your body, across to the left-hand side of your body to pick up the dumbbell, before dragging it across to the right side of your body. Put your right palm back onto the ground before repeating the movement on the other side.

Common Mistakes

Not Knowing Your Pain Triggers

If you currently have lower back pain, then the last thing you need is to go to the gym and begin an intense workout, moving around with the view that any type of exercise is beneficial. This is not a smart plan. A more practical plan would be to start understanding what triggers your back pain.

Create a pain trigger list, noting down how your back feels after, during, and before your workout. By creating a habit of marking your pain levels, you will be able to understand it better and plan your workouts to avoid pain.

Not Warming up Before Your Workout

If you don't warm up before you train, then it can create new injuries or worsen ones you already have. When your muscles stay dormant, or you don't warm them up well, you will become inflexible and stiff, which causes tears and strains. Always behind any session with some stretches.

Not Stretching Adequately or at All Before Working Out

You are able to prevent injuries by strengthening your core. However, that might not be enough. You should also undertake full-body stretching at the end of each workout and also separately to your training sessions.

Beginning With Heavy Weights

A lot of injuries occur when someone has lifted weights that are too heavy for them. While it is good to challenge your limits, you should do so in small stages gradually over time.

Using Improper Form

One of the main reasons for back pain is due to poor form. Having a curved back when you are lifting is an extremely common mistake. Overarching your back the other way is also a way you can become injured.

Always make sure you have a straight back when you are lifting, and try not to sink your hips when doing press-ups.

Chapter 3: Leg Day

Most of the muscles that you will find in your legs are considered to be long muscles. They are named this way as they stretch significantly long distances. As the leg muscles begin to relax and contract, they shift the skeletal bones to make the movement of the body. Smaller muscles aid the larger muscles by stabilizing joints, rotating joints, and facilitating other movements.

The biggest muscle masses in your legs can be found in the calf and the thigh. When it comes to the leanest and strongest muscles, these can be found in your quadriceps. The four muscles that make up the quadriceps are at the front of your thigh are the major extensors of your knee, which lets you straighten your leg. They are known as;

Vastus Lateralis

Located on the outside of your thigh, this is the largest muscle out of the quadriceps. It runs from the kneecap up to the top of your femur.

Vastus Medialis

Shaped like a teardrop, the vastus medialis is on the inner thigh attached down the femur all the way down to the inner border of your kneecap.

Vastus Intermedius

Between these two muscles sits the vastus intermedius, located at the front of the femur. This is the deepest quadricep muscle.

Rectus Femoris

Finally, we have the rectus femoris, which attaches to your kneecap. Out of all of the quadricep muscles, this one has the least impact on the flexion of your knee.

Your hamstrings are made up of three muscles at the back of your thigh that impact movement at the knee and at the thigh. They start underneath your gluteus maximus, just behind your hip bone, and connect to your tibia at the knee.

Biceps Femoris

The bicep femoris is the long muscle that allows your knee to flex. It starts in the thigh region and extends all the way to the head of your fibula, close to the knee.

Semimembranosus

The semimembranosus is the long muscle that runs up from your tibia all the way to your pelvis. It helps flex the knee and extend your thigh, as well as rotating your tibia.

Semitendinosus

The semitendinosus also extends the thigh and helps flex your knee.

Our calf muscles are absolutely vital for the movement of your toes, feet, and ankles. Some of the important muscles in your calf include:

Gastrocnemius

One of the biggest muscles in your leg, which connects at your heel. It extends and flexes your feet, ankles, and knees.

Soleus

The soleus runs all the way from the heel to the back of the knee and is an essential muscle for standing and being able to walk.

Potentially one of the most important tendons when it comes to mobility is your Achilles tendon. This tendon is found at the back of the calf and ankle and links together with your gastrocnemius, soleus muscles, and plantaris to your heel bone. The Achilles tendon holds the energy you need to jump, run, and complete other physical activity.

Different Exercises for Training Legs

In the Gym

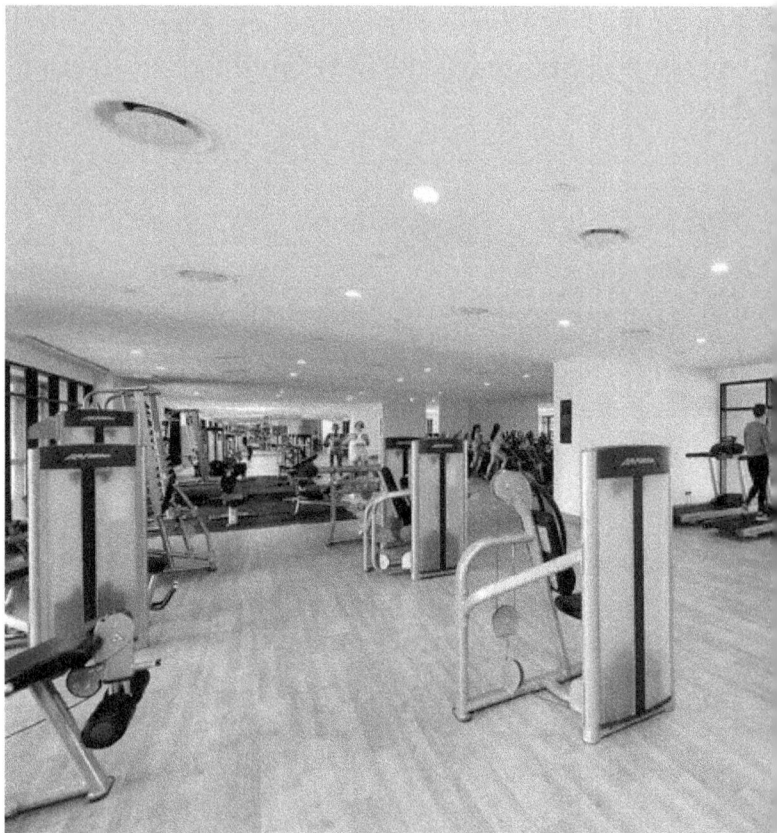

Dumbbell Step Up

Station yourself standing behind a bench or a different similar elevated surface that will place your thigh parallel to the floor when you place your foot on it. Grip a dumbbell in both hands, and then step up onto the bench, leaving your trailing leg hanging off the side.

Deadlift

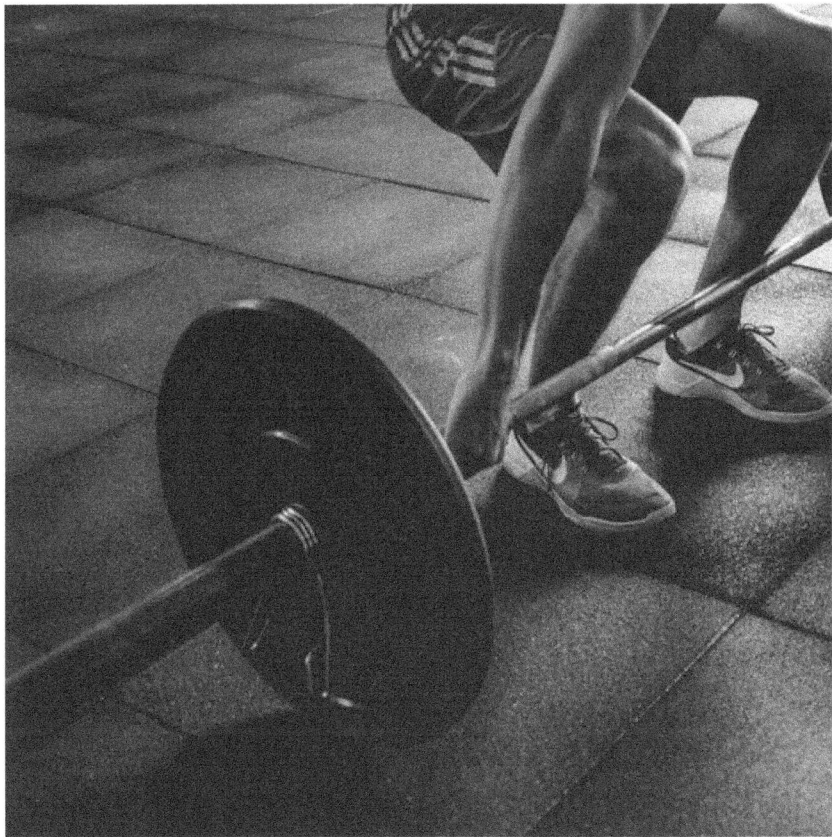

Stand upright with your feet shoulder-width apart and each shin one inch from the barbell. Grab the bar with either reverse or normal grip, bend your knees before pushing them into your arms, which should be straight.

Bring the chest up as much as you can, maintaining your gaze directly ahead. Keep your back flat before extending your hips, allowing you to stand up. As you do, pull the back up close to your legs to lockout.

Swiss Ball Leg Curl

Place your heels on the ball for stability, and then brace your abs. Raise your hips up into the air, making sure that you keep your legs straight. From that position, bend your knees to bring the ball back towards your bottom. Make sure that you keep elevated hips throughout every set.

Single-Leg Romanian Deadlift

Keep a dumbbell held in one hand and stand on one leg, the opposite one from the hand holding the weight. Bend your hips back and start to lower your torso until you feel as though your back is going to lose its arch. Tense your glutes and fully extend your hips to come back up.

Leg Press

Change the seat of the leg press machine to ensure that you can sit on it comfortably and that yours are beneath your knees, with your knees in line with each foot. Take the safeties off and lower your knees down to your chest until you hit 90 degrees before pressing back up to complete the repetition. Make sure that you don't go too low. Otherwise, you will risk your lower back breaking contact from the seat, which could cause you some serious injury.

Bodyweight Calf Raise

Place your toes on the end of a block or step and put your hand onto something sturdy for grip and support. Begin by raising your heels so that you end up on the balls of your feet before lowering your heels down until you start to feel a stretch in each calf.

Walking Lunge

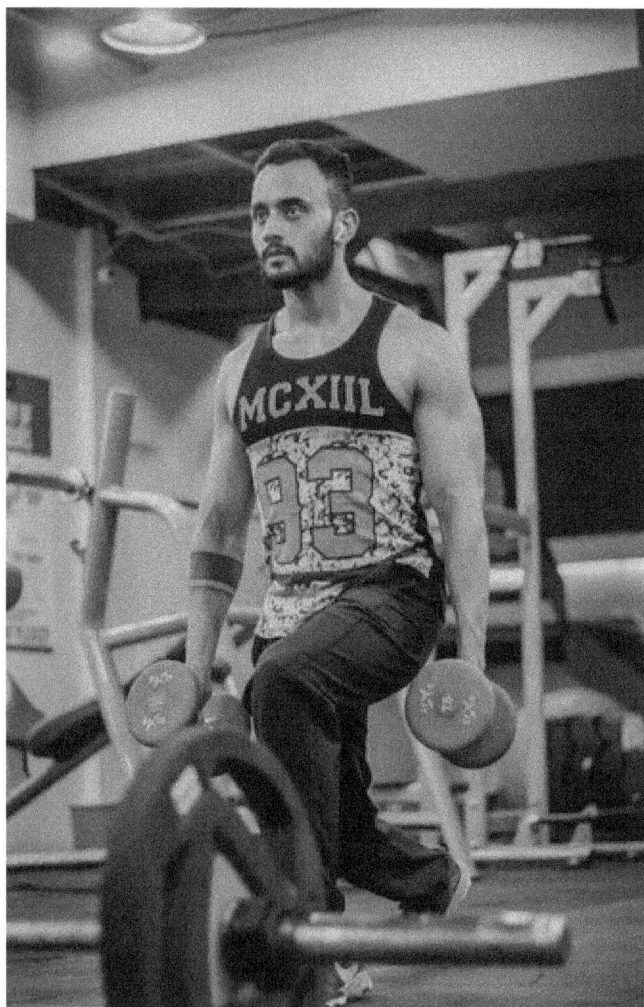

Place your feet shoulder width apart, gripping a dumbbell in each of your hands. Step forward with your left leg, lowering your body until your back knee is touching the floor and the thigh of your front becomes parallel with the floor. Step forward with your back leg and perform again on the opposite side.

Pause Squat

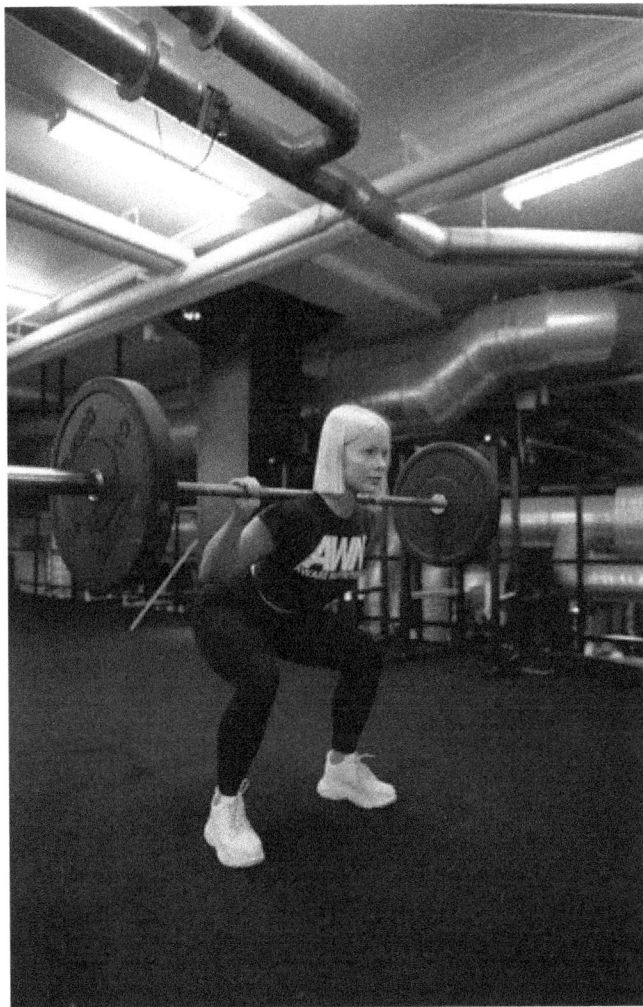

Set yourself up in a cage or squat rack. Grab the bar slightly wider than shoulder-width apart and then step under it. Tense your shoulder blades and squeeze them together before nudging the bar out of the rack. Step backward and stand yourself with your feet shoulder-width apart and with your toes slightly turned out. Inhale deeply and tuck your hips back before bending your knees to bring your body down as far as possible without losing your lower back arch. As you descend, push your knees out, and then hold for two seconds at the bottom of the squat.

Reverse Lunge

Stand with two dumbbells in your hands before stepping backward with your left foot. Lower your body down until your front thigh becomes parallel to the floor and your back knee touches the floor. Keep an upright torso throughout the movement. Step forward to complete the repetition before swapping to your other leg and repeating.

Dumbbell Squat

Hold both dumbbells at shoulder height, with legs at hip-width and your feet turned out slights. Then, squat to the deepest point you can reach without losing your lower back arch before pushing back up to complete the repetition.

Kettlebell Swing

Start by standing with your feet hip-width apart and with the kettlebell sat on the floor between your legs. Grab the weight with both hands, making sure both palms are facing your body. Keep your lower back flat, extend at the hips, and this will raise the weight off the floor. Take a deep breather before bending your hips backward, which in turn will allow the weight to swing backward, in between your legs. Drive your hips into extension, allowing the momentum to take the weight up towards shoulder height. Make sure that you control the descent before using the momentum to start the next rep.

At Home

Squat

Squats target your hamstrings, quads, and glutes. Stand with your feet shoulder-width apart, making sure your chest stays upright and back remains straight throughout the movement. Lower your body by bending your knees, moving your hips back until your thighs hit parallel to the floor. Push through your heels to the floor and drive up to standing.

Lunge

Lunges target your glutes, quads, and hamstrings. From a standing position, take a large step forwards with your left foot, lowering yourself down until your back knee is touching the floor and your thigh is parallel to the floor. As you may not have weights to hand, you can either upgrade these to jumping lunges or do more repetitions than you would with weights.

Pistol Squat

Pistol squats also work your hamstrings, quads, and glutes and are possibly the hardest bodyweight squat variation to master. Stand on a single leg before dropping into a full squat, sticking your raised leg out in front of you without it touching the floor.

Don't be disheartened if you can't do this; it's one of the toughest bodyweight movements.

Good Morning

Start by standing with your feet hip-width apart and your hands locked behind your head. Bend your body forwards by hinging at the hips, to the point that you feel a stretch in your hamstrings, before reversing the movement to come back up. This will work your glutes and hamstrings as a result.

Donkey Kick

Another move that you can do at home to target your hamstrings and sluts is the donkey kick. Position yourself on all fours, with your knees on the floor below your hips and your hands below your shoulders. Activate your core and lift your left leg behind you, staying bent at the knee, pushing the sole of your foot up towards the ceiling. Bring the leg back down slowly to complete the rep.

Side Lunge

Now to work, your abductors! Start in a standing position, take a large step to one side and lower yourself down until your knee of the leg you have moved is bent to 90 degrees, and your other leg remains straight. Push back to standing to complete the repetition.

Glute Bridge

Another excellent leg movement for your glutes and hamstrings are glute bridges. Lie down on your back with both knees bent and your feet positioned close to your glutes. Bring your hips up so that you form a straight line with your body from your neck to your knees before lowering back down slowly.

Stiff-leg Deadlift

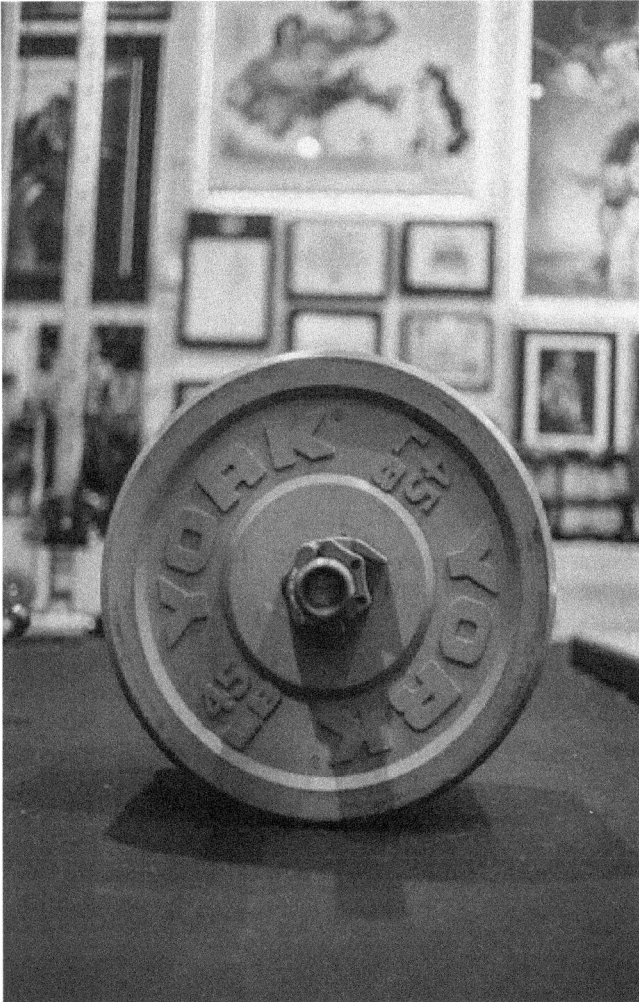

This one will need you to find a form of weight to complete, whether that be a couple of dumbbells or your own DIY alternative. Stand holding one of the weights in each hand while keeping your knees slightly bent. Keep that bend in your knees all the way through the movement. Bend at your hips to lower the weights, keeping them near your legs and ensuring your back stays straight. Once you feel the stretch through your hamstrings, slowly straighten yourself back up.

Exercises to Avoid and Why

Many people don't look forward to training legs. Leg workouts are often a bit more challenging, especially as we spend a lot of our day sitting behind a desk in most jobs. Almost all of our modern-day life revolves around being sat and not actively moving, often getting around via vehicle rather than by foot. We sit at our desks, we sit in traffic in our cars, and often our posture while we sit awful.

We hunch over our keyboards, and we hunch over our smartphones. The results from all this sitting and being hunched over is that glutes become very tight, as do our hamstrings and hips. All of these factors lead to exercising legs becoming very tough. Here are a few exercises that you need to take off your workout list to ensure you don't experience any unnecessary pain or injuries.

Leg Extension

When you extend your knees, you place a significant amount of tension on your ACL, and all you are really achieving in return is isolation in the quads. Instead, focus on other moves such as step-ups. They challenge the quads using a stepping motion, which better mirrors movements you do in everyday life.

Box Jump

We've all seen the horror videos of people failing to land a jump and falling off the box, either onto their face or into other people or equipment. I'm a big advocate for building explosive power, but it isn't the safest way to achieve those types of results.

Instead, look at trying out squat jumps rather than box jumps. Squat jumps for you to focus on your ankles, knees, and hips. This triple flexion response builds power in your jump, without the chance of creating an injury in the process.

Thigh Machine

Aside from the fact that you look silly and might strain your knees with this machine, it also isn't an effective way to test your hip adduction and abduction. Resistance bands are much more effective for working these muscles. Wrap one around both legs just on top of your knees. For a mid squat position, keep your right leg stationary, then rotate your left knee in and out. Switch legs and repeat.

Weighted Step Ups

Apart from getting in the way of other gym users, walking up and down the steps of your gym with dumbbells in your hands places undue strain on your knees. Instead, try a farmers walk. It is a great exercise that provides similar benefits, but without placing pressure on your knees and the added benefit of building your core and improving your posture.

Common Mistakes

Forgetting to Focus on Form

Not focusing on form and focusing on heavyweights instead can cause major injury issues. Pointing your toes out slightly will work your outer quads more in a squat. It is essential to focus on form and ensure you are working the right areas when training legs to avoid injuries.

Stretch Before and After

If you are suffering from any pain, such as in your knee, you may feel as though you need to take a few days off, but this may not be the case. Tight muscles of the hips could be the reason you are experiencing this pain, which tends to come from not properly stretching before and after a leg workout. Leg workouts can lead to pain and aches if you don't stretch properly, making sure you focus on your hips just as much as other areas.

Using weight That is too Heavy

Of course, there are few better feelings in the gym than lifting heavier than you have done before, but you need to be realistic with how much weight you're lifting, ensuring you keep proper form. Putting too much weight on the bar may stop you from being able to complete a full range of motion per rep. While you might be able to go up in weight, if you can't complete the full range, then you will need to build up until you can.

Chapter 4: Abs

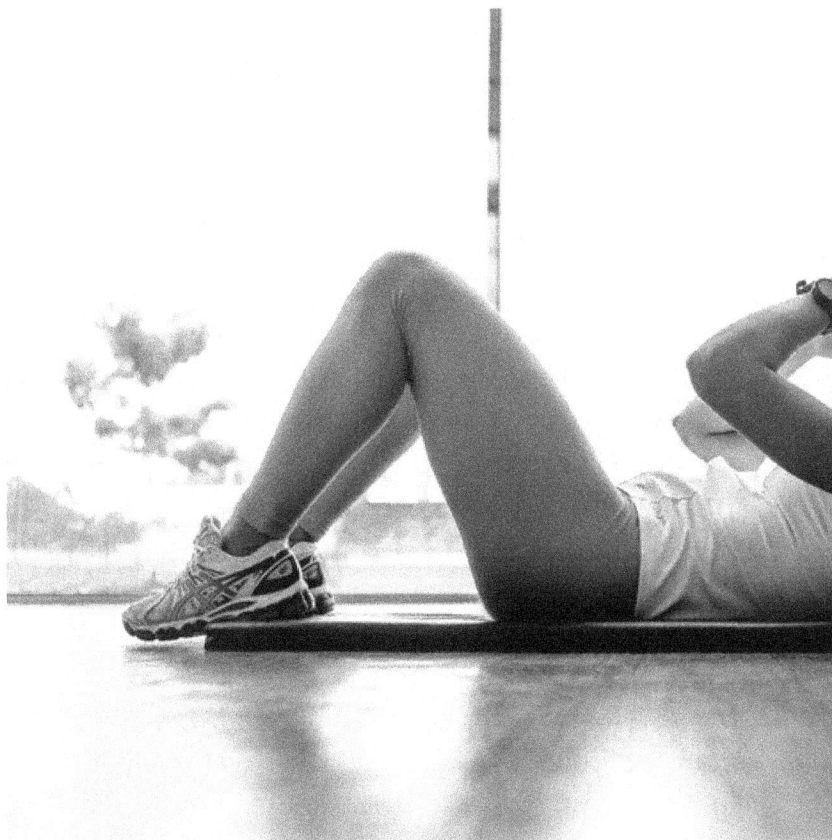

Your abdominal muscles can be found in between your ribs and your pelvis, at the front of your body. Your abdominal muscles help support your trunk, which allows you to move and holds organs in the right place by regulating and maintaining internal abdominal pressure.

Abdominal Muscles Explained

The four most important abdominal muscle groups that merge to completely cover your internal organs include:

Transversus Abdominis

This is the deepest muscle layer, and it's main roles are to ensure your trunk is stabilized and keep internal abdominal pressure.

Rectus Abdominis

Found in between your pubic bone and your ribs at the front of your pelvis, when the rectus abdominis contracts, this muscle creates the bumps that are referred to as a six-pack. The main function of this muscle is to shift the body in between your pelvis and ribcage.

External Oblique Muscles

Your external oblique muscles can be found on each side of your rectus abdominis. These muscles allow you to twist your trunk.

Internal Oblique Muscles

The internal oblique muscles flank your rectus abdominis and can be found just inside your hip bones. These muscles operate in the exact opposite way to your external oblique muscles.

Core Muscles

Try to imagine your core as a strong column that links together with your lower body and upper body. Having a strong core provides you with the foundation to complete any activity. All of the movements we make are powered by our torso, with the back and abdominals working together to help support our spine when we exercise, pick things up, bend over, stand, or even sit.

Your core muscles are located deep inside your back and abdominals, attaching to the pelvis or spine. A few of these muscles include your transversus abdominis, which are the muscles of your pelvic floor, and your oblique muscles.

Another muscle that is essential in moving your trunk is the multifidus. This muscle sits deep in your back and runs along your spine. It works in collaboration with your transversus abdominis to improve spine stability and work at preventing back strain or injury as you move or even within your normal posture.

Different Exercises for the Abs

In the Gym

I'm a big fan of bodyweight movements, such as the plan and the benefits that they bring to your core. In fact, you likely have a number of bodyweight exercises that you try when you are looking to work your core.

But have you ever considered working your abs using the equipment you can find in your local gym? I have lined up some killer core exercises, using some of the more common equipment that you can find in most gyms.

Next time you are in the gym and don't fancy doing yet another crunch, choose a couple of the moves highlighted in this chapter for two or three sets, and you're guaranteed to feel the burn pretty quickly!

Hanging Leg Circles

Grab a pull-up bar with your arms extended and palms parallel. The bar needs to be high enough that you are able to hand it with extended legs, without your feet being in contact with the floor. Engage your core and keep your legs straight before drawing a large circle in the air with your toes.

Make sure that you brace your abs tightly, which will stop you swinging back and forth, before reversing the circle.

Hanging Bicycles

This one can make it look like you are trying to run in the air, but the results speak for themselves! Grab a pull-up bar with your arms extended and your palms parallel. Engage your core and bring your knees up to around a 90-degree angle, ensuring your thighs run parallel to the floor. From that position, pedal your flexed feet, like you would if you were riding a bike.

Maintain controlled movements for 30 seconds if you can.

Hanging Side-to-side Knees

Another core exercise for utilizing the pull-up bar. Grab it, extend your arms, and ensure your palms are parallel. Engage your core before lifting your knees to the left side of your torso, letting your legs bend at the knee. Bring your knees as close as possible to the right-hand side of your chest before lowering back down to the starting position and repeating on the other side.

Cable Isometric Hold

Don't be intimidated by the cable machine! It is much easier to use than you might think. Start by stacking a lightweight before positioning the carriage so that it is level with your chest. Then stand alongside the machine, with your right side facing away from it.

Next, grab one cable handle with both of your hands. Take a large step away from the cable machine, and extend both of your arms out in front of you at chest height. Drop into a half-squat position, holding the weight steady.

Engage your abs and grip the handle directly in front of you; don't allow your body to turn towards the machine. Hold for half a minute, and then switch sides.

Cable Oblique Crunch

Stack a medium weight on your cable machine and move the carriage down to the setting that is closest to the floor. Standing with your left side perpendicular to the cables, grab a cable hand in your left hand. Place your right hand behind your head.

Next, engage your obliques and lean to the right, away from the cable machine, essentially performing a side crunch but in a standing position. Return to the starting position before completing a few reps and swapping sides.

Side Plank With Cable Hold

Making sure that you have already mastered the bodyweight side plan, then you will be good to try out this one. Load a lighter weight onto the cable machine, moving the carriage down to the bottom setting, and positioning yourself a couple of feet away from the cables.

Grav the cable in your right hand and come into a side plant on your left forearm, bracing your core and stacking your feet. Extend your right arm so that your body comes into a T shape. Hold for half a minute and then swap sides.

Overhead Kneeling Cable Hold

Place a light load on the cable machine before sliding the carriage down to the lowest setting, nearest the floor. Start with the left side of your body facing the machine, with your left foot and right knee touching the floor.

Hold a cable handle in both hands before pulling it overhead, using your hands to maintain the overhead position of the cable. The aim is to stay perfectly straight, keeping your core engaged.

Hold this position for 30 seconds before repeating on the other side.

At Home

Abs Workout One: Unilateral Powerhouse

This exercise set is excellent for targeting your deep core muscles and promotes good posture. Complete three rounds of this workout:

1. 15 Dumbbell Renegade Rows

2. 15 Single-Arm Dumbbell Overhead Press and a twist on each side

3. 8 Split Squats on each side

4. 20 Dumbbell Suitcase Walking Lunges on each side

5. 8 Single-leg Squats and a Dumbbell Lateral Raise, with weight in the hand of your working leg.

6. 15 Single-leg Deadlift

7. Side plank with ten dumbbell flyes on each side

Abs Workout Two: No-crunch Workout

In this workout, there is so much stabilization required that your whole core will be burning far more than it would after doing one hundred crunches.

Do three rounds of:

1. 30 Lying Bicycle Crunches holding a dumbbell overhead, not touching the ground

2. 10 Press-ups

3. 1-minute Side Plank

4. 1 minute Front Plank

5. Side Plank with 15 Dumbbell Flyes (each side)

Abs Workout Three: Cardio Core Shred

Get the blood pumping with this spicy abs workout! Three rounds of the following circuit, with one-minute rest in between, is sure to get those calories burning!

1. 18 Skater Lunges

2. 18 Mountain Climbers

3. 18 Burpees

4. 18 Knee-to-Shoulder Knee-ins, switching sides after each rep

5. 1-minute Side Planks

Abs Workout Four: Plank Variations

Staying still in a basic forearm plank for ages is not only boring but also extremely counter-productive as a lot of people tend to lose their form after the first minute, creating too much strain on their backs.

Instead, this routine keeps you switching and moving around, so you get the same benefits, if not more, without any of the unnecessary back pain. Added bonus, you don't need any equipment to do this workout!

Complete this plank series a couple of times, taking adequate rest in between rounds:

1. 12 Forearm Side Planks

2. 12 Press-ups into a Straight-arm Side Plank

3. 1-minute Side Plank

4. Normal Planks with 18 Toe Taps, completing nine on one side and then nine on the other side

5. Forearm Plank with 18 Side-to-Side Hip Dips

6. 18 Knee-to-Shoulder Knee-ins

7. 18 Knee-to-Opposite-Shoulder Knee-ins

8. 12 Forearm Side Planks

Abs Workout Five: Standing abs Workout

Not all of your core work has to be completed lying down. Aim for three rounds of the following circuit, with no rest in between.

1. 18 Dumbbell Chops, 18 on each side

2. Plank with 24 Knee-ins, both knees counts as one rep

3. 10 Forward Lunges

4. 10 Single-leg Squats

5. 10 Dumbbell Overhead Press

6. 8 Dumbbell Swings

Abs Workout Six: Bodyweight abs Workout

Don't have access to any equipment? Have no fear. Complete three rounds of this circuit as fast as you can, making sure to keep good form throughout:

1. 24 Butterfly Kicks, completed lying on your back

2. 24 Crunches

3. 24 Russian Twists

4. 24 Elbow-to-Knee Crunches

5. 24 Butterfly Sit Ups

6. 24 Crunches

7. 24 Butterfly Kicks, completed lying on your back

Abs Workout Seven: Anti-flexion Workout

These exercises work by making your body resist flexing forwards, ensuring that your core muscles remain more stable. Complete three rounds of the following:

1. 18 Supermans

2. 18 Dumbbell Pullovers

3. Forearm Planks with 18 Toe Taps on each side

4. Side Planks with 18 Leg Pendulums on each side

5. 24 Prone Reverse Crunches

6. Side Plank with 18 Dumbbell Flyes each side

7. 1-minute Forearm Plank

8. 18 Supermans

Abs Workout Eight: Deep V Workout

The objective of this workout is to sculpt the V shape into your abs. Complete four rounds of this circuit:

1. 16 Lying Alternating Leg Lifts (each side)

2. 18 Supine Reverse Crunches with Overhead Dumbbell

3. 24 Bicycle Crunches

4. 12 Inchworms

5. 18 Knee-to-Shoulder Knee-ins

6. 18 Knee-to-Opposite-Shoulder Knee-ins

Abs Workout Nine: 5-minute abs Circuit

When you are a little short for time to train but still keep to get a workout in, then you can complete anywhere between three to five rounds of this circuit:

1. 18 Dumbbell Pullovers

2. 24 Bicycles with Full Leg Extension

3. 1-minute Forearm Plank followed by 20 Side-to-Side Hip Dips

Abs Workout Ten: Rotational Power Workout

Twisting, or figuring out how to counteract the twist, is a more advanced technique, but one that is very important when you are looking to improve your core power. Once you have warmed up, complete two rounds of this circuit.

1. 10 Forward Lunges with Dumbbell Twist

2. 16 Dumbbell Overhead Press with a twist

3. 24 Dumbbell Renegade Rows

4. 8 Press-ups into a Straight-arm Side Plank

5. 16 Forearm Side Plank

6. 18 Dumbbell Chops

7. 12 Side-to-side Dumbbell Chops

Common Mistakes When Training Abs

Sitting all the way up

When you are doing a standard sit-up, try not to sit all the way up. Doing this can lead to stress on your back and may require you to take a few days off training. Instead, focus on doing crunches that lift your upper body halfway up to get perfectly toned abs.

Training Every Single day

When you allow your muscles the opportunity to rest in between workouts, you will be able to train more effectively and achieve better results. Equally, the rest period will allow your body to gain strength. You should look to work different muscle groups each day to ensure you are giving your body adequate rest time.

Doing Planks for too Long

If you have excellent core muscles, then you may be able to spend large chunks of time in the plank position before you even feel a strain on your abs. Instead of upping the amount of time you spend in the plank position, look to remove one of your contact points from the ground, such as lifting one leg or one arm and then holding that position.

Expecting a Flat Stomach

Simply training your abs will not be enough for you to drop stomach fat. You can build a six-pack by doing ab exercises, but you will still be required to shed the surrounding fat. This fact doesn't get shifted by just training abs. Cardio training is also needed to help you drop those extra pounds and lose weight quicker.

Getting Stuck in the Same Routine

If you aren't careful, it can be very easy, getting too comfortable with a workout program, and you will start to lose some of your gains as a result. You should look to change up your routine now and then to keep this fresh, work new muscles, and keep yourself motivated with your training.

Not Keeping Your Stomach Flat

Training your abs is tricky and precise business. To make sure that your stomach remains toned and flat, you will need to pull in your body as you are completing ab exercises. That way, you will train your muscle memory correctly, and your stomach size will begin to drop.

Using a ball that is not fully inflated

If the ball is not fully inflated, it will flatten as you begin to curl up, making the workout less effective on your abdominal muscles. You should check to make sure that when the ball is pushed, it concaves no more than a couple of inches.

Neglecting Your Back Muscles

Exercising your abs without also training your back will lead to an imbalance in your musculature, which supports your spine. After all, these muscles aren't just for show. The best exercises to work your abdominal muscles are the ones that make your whole core work hard to support your spine as well.

Placing Your Hands Behind Your Neck

It is the belief of some people that if they put their hands on the back of their head, then they will get more support when they do sit-ups or crunches. However, this can cause serious neck injuries if you happen to pull on your neck or strain it. It also decreased the effectiveness and tension of the exercise on your abs.

Instead, look to place your hands across your chest or at your ears.

Raising your legs without any support

Trying to complete an exercise without any support can be quite counter-productive. With this exercise, which focuses on working your lower abs, it is very common for people to simply raise their legs. There are plenty of much more effective pieces of equipment to do this at the gym. These machines will support your back and help you work out the right areas. So get rid of lying on the gym floor and move to do curl-ups and the machines!

Pushing Your Bum out When Doing Planks

Performing your planks in the incorrect form will have almost no effect on working your abs. It is so easy to do planks incorrectly, as you might not even know that you are making this mistake. Having said that, it is also simple to correct once you understand how they should be done. Rather than bending over your lower back and sticking your butt up, your body should make up one line. Your spine should be straight and in line with your butt.

Chapter 5: Hands

Your hand muscles can be split into two distinct groups: your extrinsic hand muscles and your intrinsic hand muscle. The extrinsic muscles can be found in the posterior and anterior compartments of your forearm. They are in charge of crude movements and allow you to create a forceful grip. The intrinsic muscles of your hand can be found within the actual hand itself. They are required to complete any fine motor functions with your hand. In this chapter, we will focus specifically on your hand muscles, their names, and what their functions are.

Thenar Muscles

The three short muscles that can be found in the base of your thumb are the thenar muscles. The muscle bellies create a bulge, referred to as the thenar eminence. These muscles are in charge of the fine movements of your thumb. Each of the thinner muscles is innervated by the median nerve.

Opponens Pollicis

The largest thenar muscle is the opponens pollicis, which sits beneath the other two. It originates out of the tubercle of your trapezium, and the relevant flexor retinaculum goes into your lateral margin of the thumb's metacarpal.

This muscle allows you to oppose your thumbs by rotation medially and flexing your metacarpal on the trapezium.

Abductor Pollicis Brevis

The abductor pollicis brevis can be found proximal to your flexor pollicis brevis and anteriorly to your opponens pollicis. It derives from the tubercles of the trapezium and the scaphoid and via the associated flexor retinaculum. It is attached to the lateral side of the proximal phalanx of your thumb. This muscle is used to abduct your thumb.

Flexor Pollicis Brevis

The most distal thenar muscle is the flexor pollicis brevis. It attaches from the tubercle of your trapezium and the associated flexor retinaculum. It is also attached to the base of the proximal phalanx of your thumb.

This muscle flexes your metacarpophalangeal joint in your thumb.

Hypothenar Muscles

The hypothenar muscles create the hypothenar eminence, which is a muscular protrusion that is found on the medial side of your palm, located at the bottom of your little finger. These muscles are not dissimilar to your thenar muscles.

Opponens Digiti Minimi

Your opponens digiti minimi can be found deeper than the other hypothenar muscles. It starts at the hook of the hamate, and the associated flexor retinaculum. It inserts into the metacarpal V via the medial margin. This muscle allows you to rotate your little finger inward towards your palm.

Abductor Digiti Minimi

The abductor digiti minimi is the most superficial hypothenar muscle. It starts at the pisiform as well as the tendon of your flexor carpi ulnaris. It is attached to the bottom of the proximal phalanx of your little finger and helps abduct it.

Lumbricals

In total, there are four lumbricals in your hand, each associated with one of the fingers. They are essential to finger movement and link the flexor tendons and the extensor tendons. Denervation of such muscles is the foundation for the hand of benediction and ulnar claw.

All four of the lumbrical begin from a tendon that is attached to the flexor digitorum profundus. They pass laterally and dorsally around every finger and thread into the extensor hood.

Interossei

Found between the metacarpals, the interossei muscles can be split into two groups, the palmar and the dorsal interossei.

Alongside their actions of adduction and abduction of your fingers, the interossei are also on hand to help the lumbricals in their flexion and extension.

Dorsal Interossei

Out of all of the dorsal muscles, the dorsal interossei is the most superficial and can be palpated on your hand via the dorsum.

Palmar Interossei

The palmar interossei can be found anteriorly on your hand. In total, there are three palmar interossei muscles. However, some believe there to be a fourth muscle located at the base of the proximal phalanx of your thumb.

Each of the interossei starts from a lateral or medial surface of a metacarpal and is attached to the proximal phalanx or extensor hood of the same finger. These muscles adduct your fingers via the MCP joint.

Other Muscles in the Palm

There are two extra muscles in your pal that are not interossei or lumbricals, and they don't fit into the thenar or hypothenar compartments.

Palmaris Brevis

The palmaris brevis is a thin, small muscle that is located superficially inside the subcutaneous tissue of your hypothenar eminence.

The palmaris brevis starts from the flexor retinaculum and palmar aponeurosis and attached to the dermis of your skin on the medial margin of your hand. This muscle wrinkles your skin of the hypothenar eminence, which deepens the curvature of your hand, bettering your grip.

Adductor Pollicis

The adductor pollicis is a big triangular muscle that has two heads. Between the two heads, the radial artery can be found passing through anteriorly, which creates the deep palmar arch. One of the heads is attached to metacarpal III, with the other attached to the capitate and the adjacent parts of the metacarpals II and III. Both heads attach to the base of the proximal phalanx of your thumb. This muscle is the adductor of your thumb.

Different Exercises for the Hands

In The Gym

It is really important to make sure you aren't neglecting training your forearms as part of your routine. The forearms, wrists, and hands need to be focused on while warming up and also when you are working out. Here, I have highlighted some of the best wrist exercises that you can do in the gym that will let you develop strong and symmetrical forearms.

The Benefits of Forearm and Wrist Exercises

So often, people focus all of their attention on working their biceps and triceps in an attempt to get bigger arms. All the while, they neglect to train their wrists and forearms as much as they should.

Your wrists and forearms let you perform the movements that develop and increase your triceps, biceps, chest, back, and deltoid strength.

That is why it is absolutely essential for you to spend time and energy on optimizing your hand, wrist, and forearm strength.

Important Forearm and Wrist Exercises

Here are a few important tips that can really aid you in developing symmetric and strong forearms and wrists. I would suggest that you do these exercises two to three times per week.

1. Extend and flex all of your fingers while creating a complete fist for half a minute. Next, close and open your fingers—complete two sets of each of these movements.

2. Flex at the wrist and maintain in complete flex for 30 seconds, keeping your elbow straight but not fully locked out.

3. Extend the wrist keeping your elbow straight for 30 seconds. Complete two sets in two minutes.

4. Wrist Hammer Curls, Seated - In a seated position and with a straight back, lay your forearm on the thighs with both thumbs pointing upwards. Lift two dumbbells back and forth in a controlled manner for 20 reps, three times.

5. Seated Wrist Straight Curls - this exercise is designed to improve your flexor muscles. When seated, place your forearms on your thighs and point your palms upwards. With dumbbells in hand, flex your wrists to the sky. Maintain the forearm position on your thighs to get more isolation of the wrist and better stability. Make sure you place your wrist four inches away from the knee to get a full range of motion. Do 20 repetitions three times.

6. Seated Reverse Wrist Curls - This exercise helps develop your extensor muscles and is another one that is done in the seated position, with both forearms placed on your thigh, with your palms pointing downward. Make sure your wrist is four inches from your knee. Grab the weights and extend your wrist completely. Complete 20 reps for three rounds and ensure that your elbow does not move from your thigh as you extend your wrists.

7. Finger Curls - this is such a simple exercise to do and will improve your hand strength and finger strength. Sit down and place a weight in your hand. Turn the hand so that your palm is facing upward so that the back of your wrist is sat on your thigh. Let the weight turn through your finger, curling them back to keep the dumbbell in place.

From strength to precision to endurance, almost all athletes' performance will be improved through improved grip strength. At one time or another, most sports require you to hold something of some kind as part of the game. In sports that include obstacle courses or lifting heavy weights, grip strength may be the ultimate deciding factor that determines whether you win or lose.

Whatever your body weight may be, the muscles of your arms, hands, back, core, and shoulders all play a part in having the ability to squeeze or hold on to things. However, the important aspect of these muscles is not how big they are; it is how strong and how much endurance they have. Often bodybuilders can muscle their way in the gym without any grip training, but it is best to get your body ready for high grip demands to make sure you can keep lifting weights in for longer, not to mention injury prevention.

Check out these exercises that you can do to increase your grip strength.

Dumbbell Farmer's Walk With Towel

For this exercise, you will need two towels. Loop one of your towels around the handle of both of the dumbbells, and grip the ends of both towels while you stand upright and with your shoulders pinched back. Walk for fifty yards around the house or in the garden. If you are in the gym, you can use weight plates instead of dumbbells for this workout.

Dead Hang

This one requires a pull-up bar or something similar to that, which is sturdy overhead. Slightly raise your scapula to make sure your core is engaged, and your back muscles are activated. Hang onto the bar for as long as you can, aiming for at least 15 seconds.

Fat Gripz Dumbbell Curl

Any type of rubber tool that can add thickness to your dumbbells is needed for this exercise. These grip-improving tools can be used for several different strength training moves, but when you use them for biceps curls, it emphasizes the grip with every curl.

Place one of the rubber grips over each of the handles of your dumbbells, and then hold them with your palms facing forward. Start with your feet shoulder-width apart, making sure your shoulders are back and punched. Curl your dumbbells up to chin height, making sure the wrists are flat, and your psalm remains up at all times.

Barbell Shrug

You can shrug a normal barbell, dumbbells, a trap bar, or even cables on a machine to improve your grip strength, but this is definitely an exercise you should add to your workout program to improve your grip.

Grip a barbell in an overhand grip at shoulder-wide, so the bar is sitting in front of your hips, and your arms are straight. Stand gripping the barbell, ensuring your shoulders and back. While keeping your arms from bending, raise your shoulders and trap up to the ceiling, pausing for three seconds and then returning to the starting position.

Deadlift

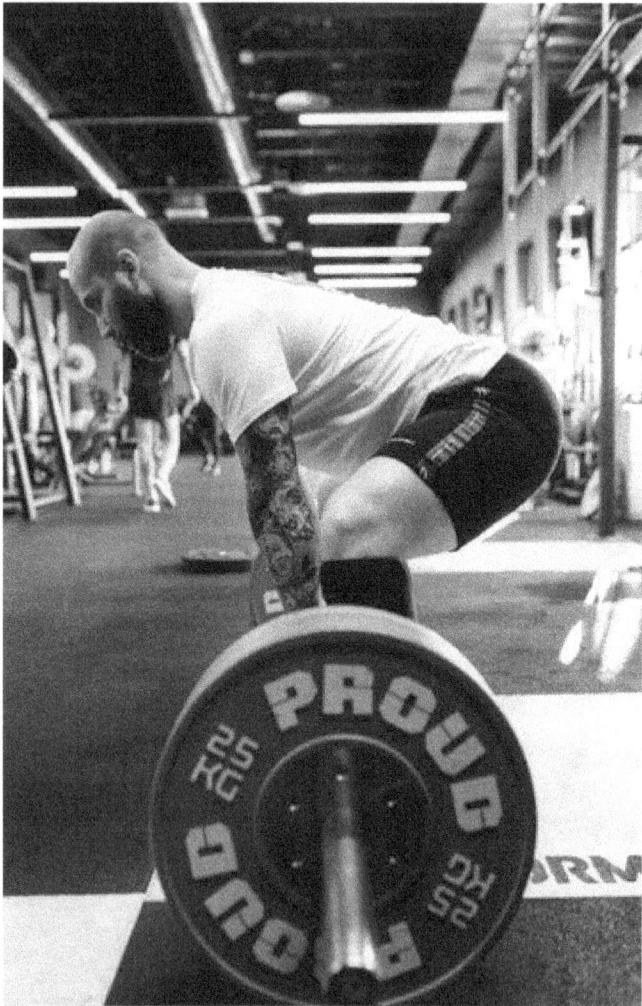

If you are deadlifting to improve your grip, then you should try deadlifting with an alternated grip. This is where you have the right hand over the top and your left hand placed in an under grip.

If the weight is becoming too heavy and you need to use a mixed grip, then your workout has changed to a strength one, and it is no longer grip focused.

Reverse Barbell Wrist Curl

This exercise is simply to improve your muscular endurance in your forearms, which in turn should transfer over to the ability to improve your lifts. Grip a barbell, a barbell in an overhand grip, behind your back. While maintaining an upright posture, allow the barbell to roll over onto your fingertips, allowing your arms to stay straight.

Then, make a fist and pull the forearms so that you can grip the bar with a closed grip.

Resisted Hand Opening

Ensure that all of your fingertips are touching each other, allowing the thumb to touch the tip of each of the fingers. Put a rubber back around the fingers and thumb before pushing your fingers out against the band, prying your hand open completely.

Pinch Grip Plate Holds

This exercise creates the ability for you to hold something for a prolonged period. Put a weighted plate flat on the floor, with a bench or a box close by. If the plate can stand on its own, then you can have it propped up. If not, rest it against the box or bench. Pick up the plate with just your left hand, using only your fingers, not including your thumb. Stand up fully with the plate in your hand, pausing for five seconds before putting it down and repeating on the other side.

How to Avoid Injury

Let's have a look at some of the most influential hand exercises that you can do daily to prevent yourself from getting injured, especially if you spend a lot of time behind a computer.

Shake It Out

Shaking your wrists and hands out after you have been in the same position for a prolonged period is an excellent way to allow blood flow to come back and remove joint stiffness. Start with both hands out in front, with your palms facing the ground. Slowly shake each hand by allowing your wrists to go limp. Repeat this three times.

Fist to Hand

The fist to hand exercise is a brilliant method to stretch out your entire hand. This allows the joints and muscles to alleviate stiffness. Start with your hands in front and your palms pointing downwards. Create a fist with each hand. Open your fist halfway until your fingers are bent on your knuckles. Hold this for two seconds. Then, fully open your hands and hold for two seconds. Repeat this five times.

Thumb Touches

Thumb touches let you improve your coordination in your forefingers and thumb, as well as enable blood flow back into the area. Hold your hands out with your palms pointing to the sky. With your left hand, bring the thumb to contact each fingertip. Repeat on both hands, five times.

Basic Wrist Stretch

This exercise is an easy and effective way to eradicate joint stiffness in your wrists, especially if you have been sitting typing for a long time. Hold your left hand out in front, with your palm facing the sky. Grip each of your fingers with your right hand. Pull your fingers down to the floor. Hold that position for ten seconds before repeating on the other side five times.

Thumb Flexion and Extension

This exercise movement is a brilliant way to focus specifically on the thumb, which can become stuff after a long day behind a desk. Start with your hands in front of your body, with each palm facing outwards. Slowly and gently extend your thumb across your palm until you start to feel a stretch. Hold that stretch for ten seconds before releasing back into the starting position. Repeat this ten times on each side.

Wrist Flexion and Extension

This exercise is a direct way you can tackle wrist stiffness and will help you increase the blood flow in your wrist and fend off injuries such as RSI and carpal tunnel.

Start by sitting down, with your feet planted flat on the floor. Rest your right arm on the edge of a surface, such as a desk, with the palm facing down to the ground and your whole hand resting off the edge. Stretch your hand upwards at the wrist, towards the ceiling, to the point that you can feel the stretch. Hold for 15 seconds and repeat three times before swapping hands.

Wrist Flexion and Extension II

If you are in need of a stretch that will work your entire arm, then you may want to try this one. It is great for relieving stiff joints as well. Start in a seated position, ensuring both feet are planted on the floor. Bring your arms up until they are parallel to the ground in front of you, making sure both palms are facing downwards. Bend the wrist downwards, ensuring your fingers are forming a claw. You should feel a stretch in the wrists. Hold for ten more seconds.

Flex your wrists upwards, moving the stretch into your forearms. Hold for another ten seconds and repeat the two movements five times on each hand.

Grip Strengthening

Strengthening your grip is an essential way to improve your overall forearm and hand strength. Working your grip can also improve your wrist muscle strength.

Start in a seated position, with your left arm supported by a desk or table. Hold on to a stress ball or something similar. Squeeze and then release what you are gripping using your thumb and four fingers. Repeat this fifteen times and then swap sides.

Chapter 6: The Heart

"Technique and ability alone do not get you to the top; it is the willpower that is the most important." - Junko Tabei

What is the Heart Muscle?

How have you ever sat back and wondered if the heart is classed as an organ or as a muscle? Well, this is a bit of a trick question. The heart is actually identified as a muscular organ.

An organ is a collection of tissues that work with each other to complete a specific function. When it comes to your heart, the function is to pump blood around your body.

The heart is mainly made up of a muscle tissue that is referred to as cardiac muscle. The cardiac muscle contracts as your heart beats, which in turn allows blood to go pumping through your body.

In this chapter, we will look at how heart health and cardiovascular training are essential parts of any training plan.

Anatomy of the Heart

In total, there are three layers that make up the walls of your heart. The largely cardiac muscle, the myocardium, is the middle layer. This layer is also the thickest out of the three. Cardiac muscle is a particular type of muscle tissue that you can only find in the heart. Your heart is able to pump blood through coordinated contractions of the cardiac muscle. These contractions are controlled by cells referred to as pacemaker cells.

There are four chambers inside your heart. The bottom two chambers are referred to as ventricles. These chambers pump blood around your body, which is why the walls of the ventricles are thicker and are made up of more cardiac muscle.

The top two chambers are referred to as atria. These chambers receive blood from different parts of your body.

The inside of your heart also has structures known as valves—these valves aid your blood to flow in the right direction.

What the Heart Does

Your heart is absolutely necessary for your body's overall function and health. If your heart does not execute the pumping action, then blood would not be able to pass through your circulatory system. Without this, other tissues and organs of the body wouldn't have the ability to function properly.

Blood offers the tissues and cells of your body the necessary nutrients and oxygen. On top of this, waste products such as carbon dioxide are also taken away by the blood, to be removed from the body.

Conditions That Affect the Heart

There are several conditions that will impact your heart. Let's look at some of the more common ones.

Coronary Artery Disease

Coronary artery disease occurs when your blood supply to the tissue of your heart is impacted. It takes place when plaque builds up on the artery walls. Arteries are needed to supply blood to your heart, and the plaque can narrow or even block them.

Risks that impact coronary artery disease are family history, high blood pressure, and high cholesterol.

People that have coronary heart disease become more at risk for other heart issues such as arrhythmia, heart failure, and heart attack.

Symptoms of coronary artery disease include angina, which is where you feel pressure, tightness, or pain when you do physical activity. It often starts in your chest before spreading to other places such as your back, jaw, or arms.

Other symptoms can also be things such as nervousness and fatigue. Treatment for coronary artery disease includes lifestyle changes, medications, or even surgery.

High Blood Pressure

Blood pressure is the amount of pressure that the blood pushes onto the walls of your arteries. If your blood pressure is too high, then it could become dangerous and may leave you at risk of a stroke or heart disease.

Obesity and chronic conditions such as diabetes can be significant risk factors that cause high blood pressure.

High blood pressure tends to be symptomless, so it is normally identified when you visit your doctor. It can be managed through lifestyle changes and, in some cases, medication.

Arrhythmia

An arrhythmia occurs when your heart begins to beat too quickly, too slowly, or irregularly. Arrhythmia can be caused due to high blood pressure, coronary artery disease, or even scarring or damage to heart tissue.

In some cases, arrhythmia shows no symptoms. If there are symptoms, then they could include things such as chest pain, shortness of breath, or even a fluttering sensation in your chest.

Treatments for arrhythmia are dependent on the type of arrhythmia and can include procedures or surgeries, pacemakers, or medications.

Heart Failure

Heart failure occurs when your heart is unable to pump blood as well as it needs to. Conditions that cause damage or overtax your heart can create heart failure. This includes diabetes, high blood pressure, and coronary artery disease.

The most common heart failure symptoms often include being short of breath, swelling, and feeling fatigued.

Treatment for heart failure can be dependent on how severe or what type of heart failure you have. This can include lifestyle changes, medications, or even surgery.

Heart Attack

A heart attack occurs when your blood flow is blocked from getting to the heart. Coronary artery disease tends to create heart attacks. Some of the more common warning signs are shortness of breath, the feeling of indigestion or nausea, or pressure in your chest.

A heart attack needs immediate medical attention. In a hospital, medication is often used to treat a heart attack, although in some cases, surgery might be needed as well.

Advice for Heart-healthy Living

There are a number of things you can do to maintain a healthy heart. Cutting down on sodium will help reduce the chances of high blood pressure. Also, make sure you are eating enough fruits and vegetables. These foods are an excellent source of fibers, minerals, and vitamins. Changing your protein sources can also help. Choose lean cuts of meat, fish, and plant proteins such as lentils, nuts, and soybeans.

You should also include foods that contain omega-3 fatty acids, such as walnuts, flaxseed oils, mackerel, or salmon.

Try and remove trans fats from your diets, such as cakes, cookies, or french fries. Always check food labels; they offer you vital information about sodium, fat, and calorie content.

Exercises for Cardio

In the Gym

Whether you like it or not, completing cardio workouts is a huge part of ensuring you are healthy. While there are times we could see it as a chore, the benefits of cardio workouts are undeniable.

That isn't just for losing weight. Cardio also reduces stress, improves your lung and heart health, improves your muscle density, and can even lower the chances of getting certain cancers or heart diseases.

Whether you are just beginning your cardio-fitness plan or hopping back into it after taking some time off, it can be tough to work out where you should start, especially when you need to weigh up your goals, injuries, and skill level.

Here we will take a look at some of the different cardio machines you will find in the gym and what benefits they bring you.

Treadmill

When it comes to cardio machines, arguable the simplest to understand and use is the treadmill.

With one belt to stand on, and a simple set of buttons to use to start and customize your workouts, the treadmill is a popular piece of equipment and couldn't be easier to use.

Firstly, you will want to get familiar with some of the buttons that can be found on the treadmill. Once you are ready to get running, place each leg on top of the sides of the treadmill.

Select the quick-start button, which will begin the treadmill moving at a slow speed. If you have never used a treadmill before, then start walking on the treadmill, steadily increasing the speed until you feel it is at a moderate pace.

It can be tempting to do too much on your first day, but on day one, you should stick to walking.

If you are more experienced on a treadmill, then you can advance this to running, but only if you feel comfortable doing so.

One of the main benefits of using a treadmill is the variety that is available to you. Users of any skill level, age, or body shape are able to use a treadmill to increase their endurance, shed weight, and up their cardiovascular health.

Elliptical

People often dismiss the elliptical trainer as a less beneficial version of a treadmill. Usually found in the gym near the treadmills, elliptical trainers offer a low-impact, simple to understand cardio choice. Ellipticals also have a set of buttons for you to get familiar with.

Making use of an elliptical is quite simple. It is worth noting, though, that once you step onto the pedals will begin to move instantly.

Begin by getting a firm grip on each handlebar and then step onto the machine. You'll probably see that the pedals are large, but that is a good thing and will offer more stability and safety.

Ensure that you align your feet up with the edge of the pedals to make sure you aren't straining your hips. Ensure you keep proper form by tucking your abs in, straightening your back, and bringing your pelvis forward slightly.

Next, choose either the stabilizing or stationary handlebars to hold onto. Bend your elbows slightly and start pedaling! Like with the treadmill, set off at a moderate pace, without any resistance or incline. Make sure you keep a slight bend at the knee, as locked joints can cause injury.

Once you feel more comfortable, you can try to use different resistance levels to test yourself.

Indoor Cycle

Also referred to as the stationary bike or spin bike, the indoor cycle is another highly popular option for anyone's fitness routine. As a result, you can find spin classes and cycle machines in pretty much any commercial gyms. Don't buy into the hype and get started just yet, though. There are a couple of things you should know before you do.

Firstly, preparation is key. Included in this is changing your handlebar and seat height to adjust your frame. If possible, when the pedal is closest to the floor, you need your need to be extremely close to straight.

Once you have made that change, you need to focus on getting the correct cycling height for you. Try to avoid pushing your hips too far forward or straining trying to reach the pedals with your legs. If this occurs, you need to lower your seat.

When it comes to the handlebars, you are looking for your arms to be able to stretch out and touch the handlebars at shoulder height.

Now you need to strap your feet in. It may surprise you, but cycling is so much easier and much more comfortable if you use the straps.

Now that you have adjusted and strapped in, it is time for you to get moving. You may want to shift the pedals using just your toes, but avoid this as it will lead to foot strains.

Stair Climber

The stair climber is a great indoor variation of running up and down the bleachers at your local football field. This machine is made up of upward-moving steps and a set of handrails. You can use the stair climber without the handles, but they offer you more stability and balance.

What you want to avoid doing is relying on your hands too much and putting all your weight on your hands and not your legs. This reduces how much you are using your leg muscles, and subsequently, how many calories you burn.

As with any exercise I recommend, make sure you are always checking your form and not standing completely straight. You want a slight lean forward so that neither your back nor your knees are overcompensating.

As with the other machines on this list, start slowly before moving to a more testing pace. If you notice that you are grabbing the bars to stay up, then it is set too fast.

Similar to the cycle and elliptical, this piece of equipment is brilliant for anyone that is looking for a cardio machine that is low impact but will still up to your stamina. As you burn calories, you will also be working your calves, hamstrings, bum, and quads.

At Home

You don't need to be in the gym to complete cardiovascular exercises. There are plenty of options for you to do, with little or even no equipment. Make sure to warm up for at least five minutes before beginning any exercise.

Jump Rope

Jumping ropes not only improve your cardio but also helps you develop better hand-foot coordination, body awareness, and agility.

Make sure that your jump rope is adjusted to suit your height. Stand with your feet placed on the middle of your rope, and bring the handles up to your armpits. That is the height that you are looking for. If your rope is too long, you can tie it or cut it to prevent tripping over the rope.

Aim to skip for around twenty minutes, two or three times a week.

Aerobic Strength Circuit

Anaerobic strength circuit is excellent for increasing your cardiovascular and heart health, as well as building up your strength and toning your major muscle groups. When you are taking on an aerobic strength circuit, make sure that you focus on maintaining proper form with every exercise to avoid getting injured. Allow your heart rate to stay at a moderate level all the way through the workout. If you imagine being able to keep a brief conversation while you train, that is the pace you should be going at.

Look to complete an aerobic strength circuit for fifteen minutes, three or four times a week.

In the aerobic circuit below, your heart rate will increase, and your heart health and cardiovascular will also improve. Complete each exercise for 45 seconds, with a fifteen-second break after each one, for three rounds.

- Lunges

- Squats

- Push-ups

- Dips

- Torso Twists

Running or Jogging

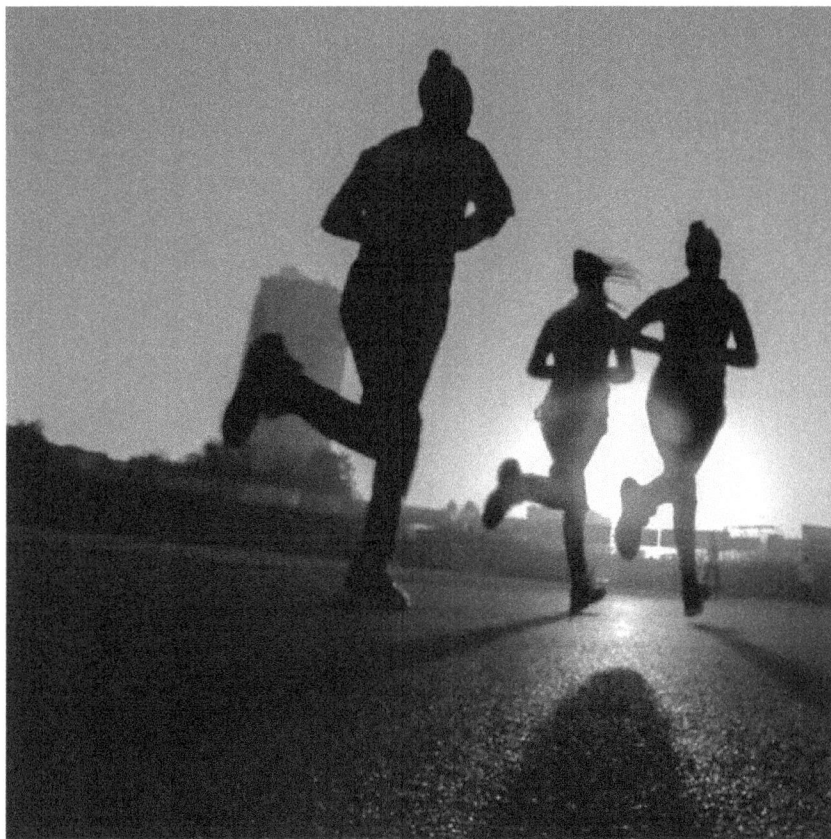

Running is one of the best types of aerobic exercise that you can do. It can increase your heart health, burn calories, and in fact, increase your mood, to name just a few benefits.

Make sure you pick somewhere you feel comfortable to go running and aim to complete a twenty to thirty-minute run, two or three times a week. If you are new to running, you can switch between running for four minutes and walking for two minutes. To make sure you prevent injuries, ensure you stretch before and after each run.

Walking

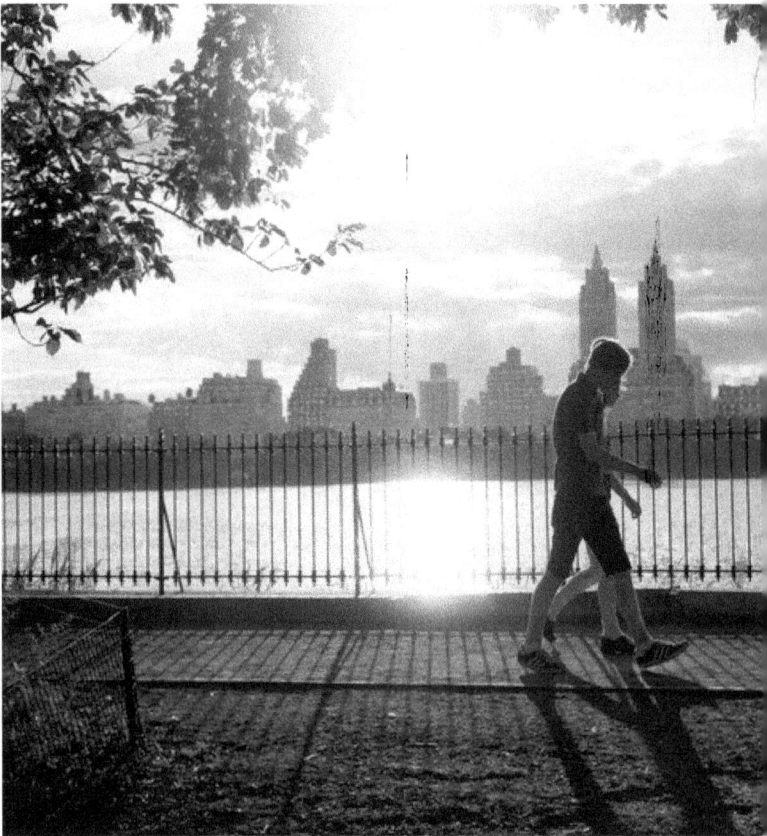

You might not know this, but walking daily is an excellent way to lower your chances of getting heart disease, diabetes, depression, high blood pressure, and obesity. If you can complete a thirty-minute walk five times a week, you will see and feel significant results.

If you like, you can take advantage of a fitness tracker to keep an eye on the number of steps you are taking every day. If you are trying to walk 10,000 steps each day, then start with a base number and slowly increase your daily steps to hit that target. You are able to do this by upping your daily steps by a further 500 steps a day each week or so.

Once you have worked out your current base number, add another 500 steps. Then, a week or two later, up your daily step count by another 500 steps.

Common Mistakes and how to Avoid Injury

Making sure your heart is in good shape is essential. That is why cardio exercises need to be a big part of your exercise plan. Here are some of the most common mistakes people tend to make when they take on cardio workouts.

Don't Use Cardio to Compensate for a bad Diet

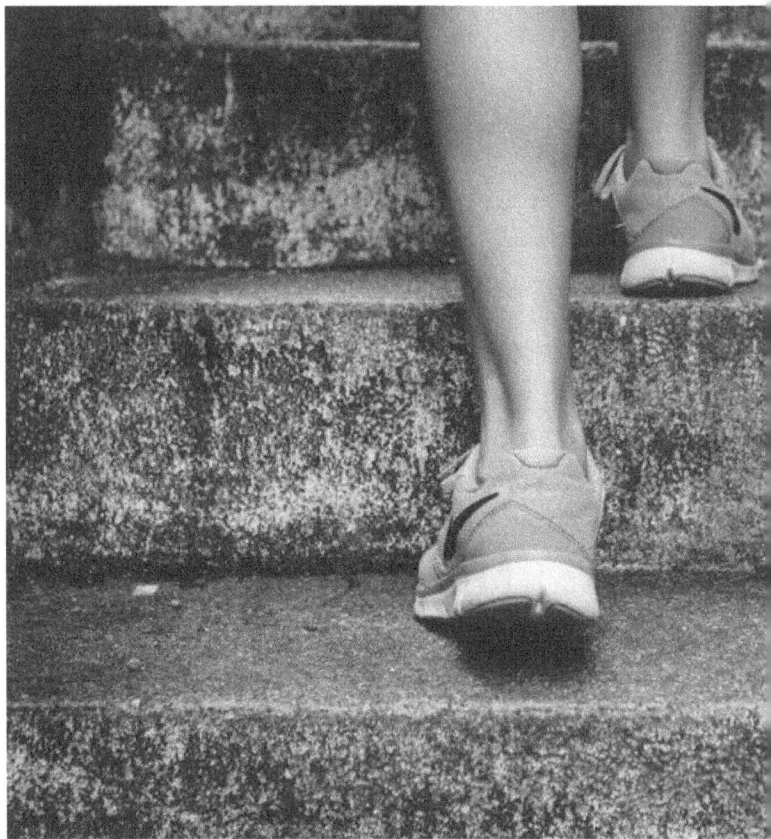

Picture this. You have spent a long time sweating your way through an intense cardio session. Then you find yourself heading to the kitchen to grab a snack. Of course, after an intense workout you need to refuel your body, but don't fall into the trap of thinking that you can eat what you want after an hour or so of cardio.

If you train with that mindset then you are likely going to have some issues with controlling your weight. Sure you can burn an impressive 400 calories in a cardio session, but you can lose that calorie deficit quickly if you reach for bad foods. You can't out-train a bad diet. Be clever, make sure to plan what food you eat, and stay on track.

Don't Overdo it

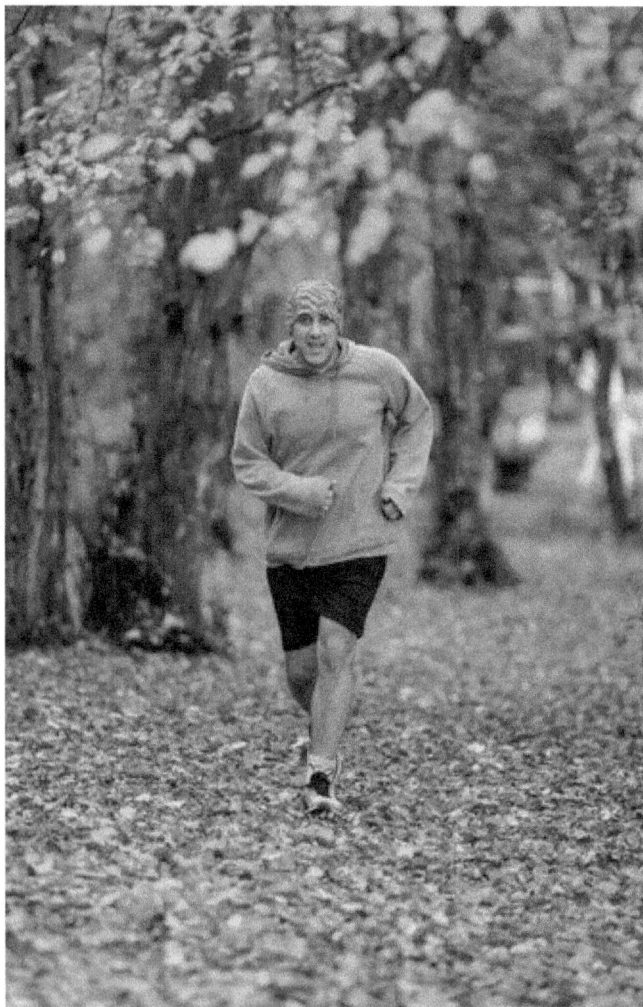

Overdoing cardio training is a common problem for a lot of people. But you don't need to follow the crowd. Devote the same amount of time to your strength workouts as you do to your cardio ones, possibly even more. Cardio doesn't influence the shape of your body. It can help you achieve weight loss, assuming that is a goal of yours, until your body changes to the stress that your cardio is achieving.

In actual fact, long periods of cardio can lead to a loss in muscle tissue if you aren't careful. If this occurs then you are actually doing more damage than good.

Vary the Intensity

Do you know anyone who tends to run the same route or complete the same treadmill or elliptical machine workout day in day out? It is likely that their weight or body composition won't change a lot over time. When you work out at the same intensity all of the time, then you aren't challenging your body to create significant results.

When you work out at a very high intensity, and then take time to recover, this activates hormones like adrenaline and growth hormone that let you drop body fat.

Mix up Your Training

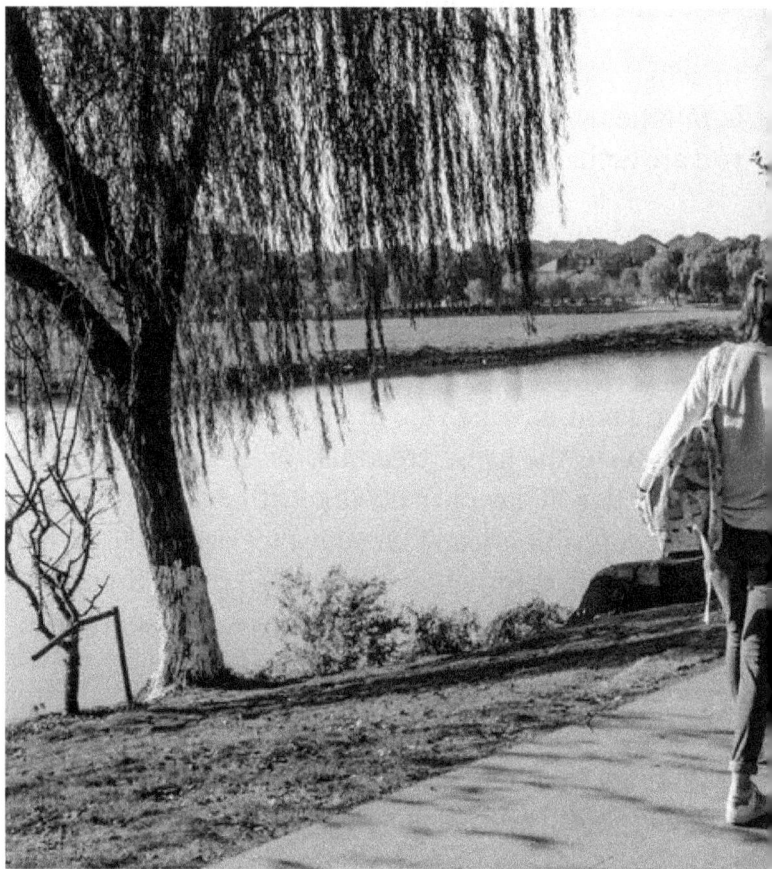

Have you ever felt stuck in a cardio rut? You can feel your eyes glazing over as you go through the motions of training. You might check the clock every couple of minutes, praying for the time to go faster.

Often people believe cardio workouts can be monotonous or boring and tend to be something that they do because they have to, and not because they want to. The truth is that cardio workouts can be monotonous if you do the same thing over and over again.

There are so many different ways that you can do cardio, so cardio ruts should never come into the equation. You can try spin or cycle workouts, kickboxing, step training, circuits, or even boot camps.

If you do the same cardio program each day, then your body becomes less efficient and each time you will burn fewer calories. Keep mixing up your training and adding variety.

Do Cardio After Weights

I'm not saying that completing cardio before lifting weights is always necessarily bad. It really depends on how long and how intense your cardio session is. If you complete an intense or long cardio session, then it is likely that you won't have enough energy to train weights properly. If you are too tired it can impact your form, and make you more susceptible to injury. To ensure you get more out of your resistance training, make sure you complete it before cardio.

Chapter 7: The Importance of Stretching

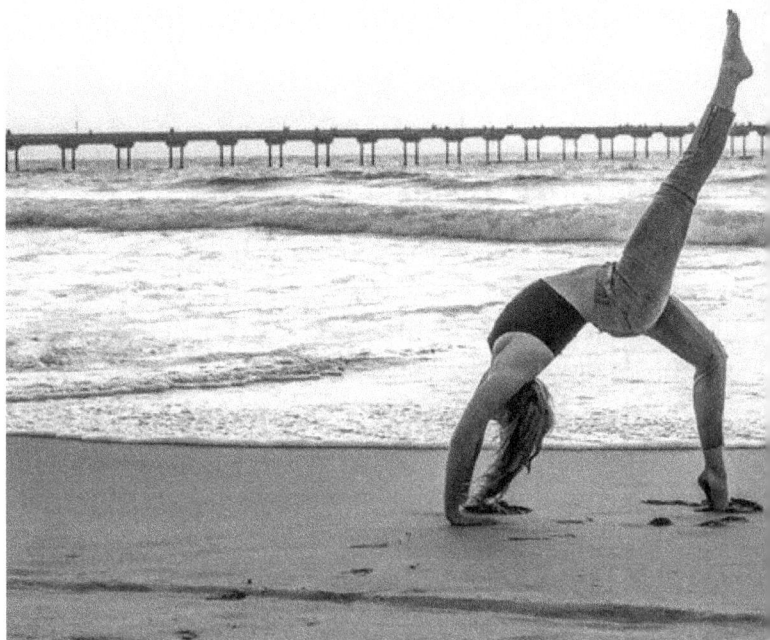

It isn't enough to simply increase your muscle and become more aerobically fit. You need to also consider your flexibility as well. That is where stretching comes into play.

You might think that stretching is something that you only need to do as an elite athlete or aspiring gymnast, but realistically we all need to stretch to make sure that we are protecting our mobility and our body.

Why Stretching is Important

Stretching makes sure that your muscles are strong, healthy, and flexible. We need this flexibility to be able to keep a range of motion in our joints. If you don't have flexibility, then the muscles will shorten and ultimately become tight. If you then need your muscles to work for you in exercise, they will be weak and will not have the ability to extend completely. That leaves you at risk of developing strains, joint pain, and even muscle damage.

For example, if you sit in a chair for a day, then your hamstrings will likely begin to tighten. This will lead to it becoming trickier to straighten your knee completely or extending your leg, which can make walking and running harder. Similarly, when you have tight muscles, and you need them to play sport or exercise, then they can become damaged from being stretched suddenly.

Stretching often allows your muscles to become lean, long, and flexible, and all this means that when you exert, then you won't be putting too much force onto your muscles.

Where to Start

Given you have a body that is packed with muscles, the concept of stretching daily can feel overwhelming. However, you don't need to stretch each and every muscle you have. The most important areas to stretch that are essential for mobility are your front of the thigh, quadriceps, pelvis, hip flexors, hamstrings, and calves. It can also be beneficial to stretch your neck, shoulders, and lower back. Look to instill a plan of stretches each day that you can complete at least three times a week.

The Cumulative Effect of Stretching

Unfortunately, simply stretching once per day will not automatically provide you with perfect flexibility. You will have to do it for a continued time period and stay committed to stretching. It can take several months to release tight muscles, so you need to bear that in mind.

Completing hamstring stretches will allow you to make sure the muscles that are in the back of your thigh stay flexible. Sit down on the floor, placing your legs out in front of you. Move your hands down your legs to the point where the back of your thighs begins to burn. Stay in that position for 30 seconds before slowly coming back up to the sitting position.

Proper Execution

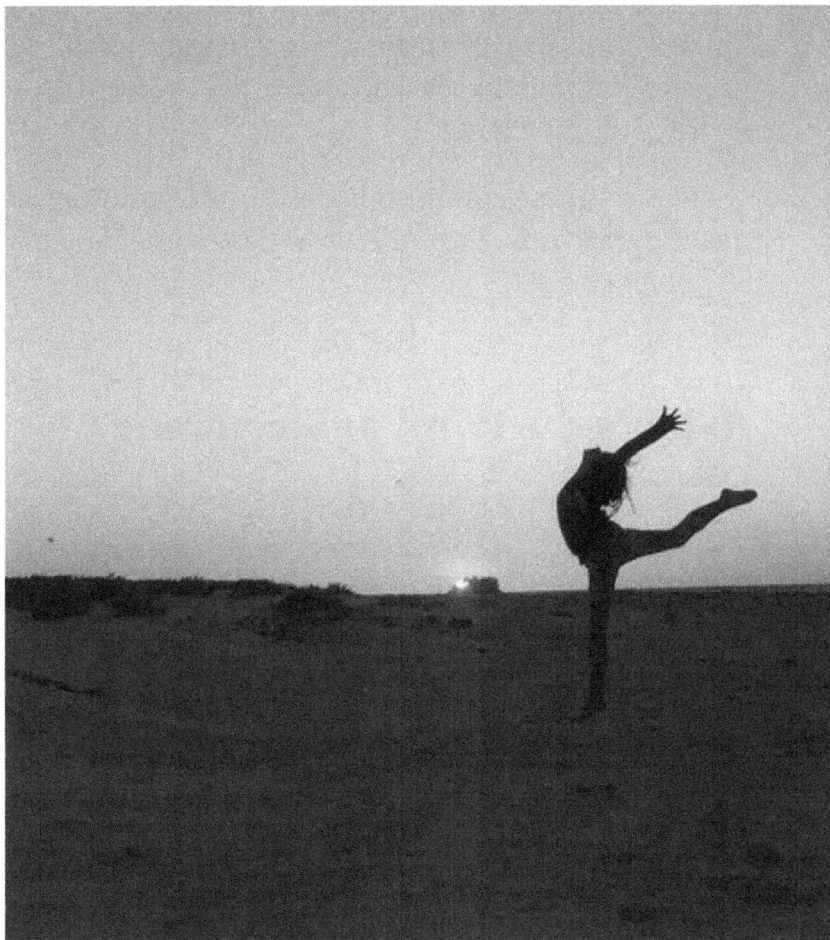

In the past, it was believed that stretching was essential to help warm up and prepare your muscles for activity. However, more and more research over time has shown that if you stretch your muscles before they are warmed up can cause more damage than good in some cases.

When your muscles are cold, the fibers are not ready for activity and could become damaged. If you get moving through exercise first, then you will allow blood flow to the muscles, which makes the muscle tissue more ready for change.

A simple warm-up of the muscles for five minutes will make a great difference and can be done through a light jog or quick walk.

What's the Point of Stretching?

Stretching for exercise and sport improves your flexibility, which improves the ability of the joint to be able to move through its entire range of motion. Essentially, that is how far the joint can twist, bend, and reach. Some physical activities, such as gymnastics, require you to be more flexible than other activities.

What Happens When We Stretch?

Although the exact mechanics of what occurs are still debated, stretching regularly is widely viewed as helping increase your flexibility by making your muscles more supple and retraining your nervous system to handle each stretch more. The flexibility you gain from stretching regularly will gradually go away if you stop stretching.

How Much Flexibility do I Need?

This all depends on what activity it is you are looking to undertake. The flexibility requirements of a gymnast compared to a runner will differ greatly. Gymnasts are likely to spend more time working on their flexibility, as it is a more important aspect of their sport.

To get the right amount of power while you are exercising, the tendons and muscles store and then release energy, much like a spring. If you are too flexible, then you could lower the muscle's natural spring, which could have a negative impact on activities such as jumping, running, or changing direction, all key components of sports like football, basketball, and baseball.

However, if your flexibility is not good enough, then this increases the chances of you getting a muscle strain injury because your muscles will be unable to lengthen enough to absorb the energy.

When do Injuries Occur?

Muscle injuries occur if you place a muscle under too much stress, often when it is put under pressure through being stretched. For example, when you are lowering down a heavyweight.

Muscle injuries occur mainly due to the muscle not being able to produce enough force to properly support itself, rather than the muscle not being flexible enough. A muscle may not be able to produce enough force, and that can be due to it not being strong enough, or it could be that the muscle didn't contract at the correct time for that particular movement.

Should I Stretch Before Exercising?

The decision on whether or not you should stretch before exercise should be based on the outcome that you are looking to achieve from that exercise. If you are trying to reduce injury, then stretching before you exercise may not be very helpful. Instead, spending time warming your muscles up through some light aerobic movements is a better option before increasing the intensity.

However, if you are trying to improve your range of motion, which in turn will allow you to move more easily, then stretching before exercise is definitely the way to go!

How Should I Warm-up?

The idea behind warming up is that you will then be physically and mentally prepared to complete the given activity. A normal warm-up will take you around ten minutes to complete and will involve some light aerobic work, topped off with a bit of dynamic stretching that mirrors some of the movements you will be performing in the upcoming activity.

As you are warming up, you should look to slowly increase the range of motion that comes for all of these movements, as that will prepare your body for the tougher version of those movements that are due to come in the workout or sport.

Warming up like this will increase your heart rate and up your blood flow into the muscles, which, as a result, will warm them up.

If your muscles are warm, then they will be less stiff, leaving them ready to work more efficiently. By increasing the blood flow, you are enabling more and more oxygen to get to the muscles, which will produce more energy. The warm-up should also be used to activate your nerve signals in the muscles, which leads to better reaction times.

Should I Stretch After Exercising?

There is plenty of evidence to show that normal static stretching that is completed outside of times when you are exercising can lead to an increase in speed and power and also lower the chance of injury. The ideal time to stretch is when all of your muscles have been suitably warmed up and are pliable.

Post-exercise stretches will also help you slow down your heart rate and breathing and take your body and mind back to their resting state.

Standing Hamstring Stretch

Stand up tall, with each foot at hip-width apart, with your knees slightly bent, and your arms by your sides. Breath in as your bend forwards at your hips, then lower your head towards the ground while making sure that your shoulders, neck, and head remain relaxed.

Next, wrap your arms across the back of your legs, and hold the stretch for at least 45 seconds before rolling your body back up once you have finished.

Piriformis Stretch

The piriformis muscle is located on the outside of your butt and is a deep internal hip rotator—the main role of this muscle to external rotation. While deep internal rotators are small, they do produce significant amounts of movement at your hip, and ten to be overlooked.

Start by sitting on the floor, with both of your legs extended out in front of you. Then cross your left leg over your right one and place your left foot flat on the floor. Place your left hand on the floor, just behind your body. Place your right hand on your left quad or your right elbow on your left knee. From there, press your left leg to the right as you turn your torso to the left.

Lunge with Spinal Twist

This stretch is absolutely vital to aid with eradicating any posture-related pain for anyone that ends up sitting down for long periods. It enables you to open up your hips and will help improve your thoracic mobility.

Begin stood up, with both feet together. Take a large step forward with your right leg, leaving you in a staggered stance position. Next, bend your right knee, which will drop you into a lung, making sure that you keep your left leg in a straight line behind you, with the toes of your left leg on the floor. This position should give you a stretch in your left thigh at the front.

Put your left hand onto the floor and begin to twist your upper body to the right as you extend your right arm up to the ceiling. Hold that position for half a minute and then repeat on the other side.

Triceps Stretch

Start by kneeling, sitting, or even standing upright, with both feet hip-width apart and your arms extended above your head. Bend your left elbow and reach your left hand to touch your upper back. Next, right your right-hand overhead and grab just under your left elbow. Slowly pull your left elbow down and in towards your head. Repeat the stretch on the other side.

Figure Four Stretch

The figure four stretch is a unique one in that it specifically stretches out your iliopsoas and piriformis muscles, as well as your IT band. Due to the passive nature of this stretch and what it helps you achieve, it is a brilliant and safe way to help relieve some of the symptoms that are associated with knee pain and sciatica.

Start by lying on your back, with your feet firmly planted on the floor. Then, cross your right foot over your left quad. Lift your left leg off of the floor. Hold onto the back of your left leg before slowly pulling it in towards your chest. When you start to feel a stretch coming on, maintain that position, holding it for at least half a minute. Switch sides and do the same again.

90/90 Stretch

This stretch is excellent for assisting with external rotation of one leg and internal rotation of the other, meaning you get both movements of your hip in one stretch. This stretch is ideal for anyone that suffers from tight hip flexors.

Start by sitting with your left knee bent at 90 degrees out in front of your body, making sure your calf is perpendicular to the body. The sole of your foot should be facing to the right. Keep your left foot flexed. Allow your leg to rest flat on the ground.

Place your right knee to the right of your body, bending your knee so that your right foot faces you. Keep your right foot flexed. Make sure you keep your left butt cheek on the floor. You want to try and move your right cheek as close as you can get it to the ground. That might not be possible if you are particularly tight. Hold the stretch for half a minute and then swap sides.

Frog Stretch

Often, we tend to sit with our legs crossed, which can result in you getting tight hips, and that can lead to lower-back issues. The frog stretch focuses specifically on right spots that can occur in your groin and hips, which is ideal for runners who tend to suffer from these issues.

Begin on all fours, sliding both of your knees slightly wider than shoulder-width apart. Point your toes out, and then rest the inside parts of your feet on the ground. Move your hips back over your heels. Shift your hands onto your forearms if you are looking for a deeper stretch, and then hold it for at least half a minute.

Butterfly Stretch

Start in a seated position, with your back upright and the soles of your feet touching each other, each knee bent out to the side. Hold onto either your ankles or your feet, begin to engage your abs, and then slowly lower your upper body down towards your feet as far as you are able while keeping your knees pressed towards the floor. If you're too stiff to bend over, then focus on bending your knees down. Hold this position for at least half a minute.

Seated Shoulder Squeeze

Sit with your knees bent on the ground, with both feet placed firmly on the floor. Clasp each hand together behind your back. Next, extend and straighten your arms, squeezing your shoulder blades together in the process. Complete this for three seconds before releasing. Repeat this six times.

Side Bend Stretch

Start by kneeling on the floor, with both legs together, an engaged core, and a straight back. Extend your right leg out to one side. Make sure your leg stays perpendicular to your body. Bring your left arm over your head, and rest your right arm on your right leg, carefully bending your torso and left arm to the right side. Make sure that your hips are facing forwards, holding the stretch for 30 seconds before repeating on the other side.

Stretching Mistakes and How to Avoid Them

Stretching is an essential component of keeping up your overall wellness. There are plenty of benefits to stretching when it is done right, such as increased flexibility and that feeling of relaxation. However, the benefits of stretching can only be experienced if you stretch properly.

It may seem straightforward to stretch but making mistakes when stretching is all too common. The poor stretching technique can create pain and injury. Make a note of these mistakes that are made all too often as you start adding stretching into your life.

Not Warming up

As I have touched on, you might see stretching as your warm-up before any type of physical exercise, but in actual fact, you should warm up before you attempt any stretching. By warming up before stretching, you will up your body's core temperature, which in turn will leave the muscles more pliable and create blood flow to each of your muscles and the connective tissue.

Any warm-up you do should be some form of light aerobic activity, such as jogging, walking, or even jumping jacks. All of these types of exercises will prepare the muscles to get stretched, and for the exercise that is due to follow, and likely to be more intense.

The aim of any warm-up is to get your heart rate rising and bring your respiratory rate up, making more blood flow. This type of activity will then loosen your muscles, adding more benefits to the stretching allowing you to avoid injuries caused when you stretch cold.

Using Improper Stretching Techniques

One other mistake that many people make when they stretch is choosing the incorrect type of stretch for what they are trying to achieve. Pick the right stretch for your activity and fitness level so that you are able to avoid the potential for injury during your workout and stretch.

Dynamic Stretching

Dynamic stretching involves going through the entire range of motion and not holding any end positions. It works by using moving stretches that mimic the movements that you are planning to perform as part of your workout. It may be beneficial to go through dynamic stretches in your warm-up as a way to prepare your muscles and joints for the upcoming static stretching.

Static Stretching

Often when people hear the term stretch, they automatically think about staying in a stretch position for a short time period. This is known as static stretching, which is performed by lengthening the muscle you are trying to stretch to the point that you notice tension and then staying in that position. Static stretches are excellent for once you have finished a workout to help alleviate muscle fatigue and lower your recovery time.

Overstretching

Stretching should never feel painful. If you exert too much energy when you stretch or go too deep into the stretch, then you may end up with a torn muscle. Make sure that you always ease into stretches slowly at first. It is common, so feel some discomfort while you are stretching, but it shouldn't ever hurt. Make sure you aren't pushing your body beyond its limitations, and make sure to always keep to a natural range of motion. If you notice tightness in a muscle area, then you should repeat the stretches a few times, making sure not to push too hard.

Bouncy Stretches

If you bounce while you are stretching too vigorously, it can lead to you getting a pulled muscle. This type of motion can make the muscle become tight to try and protect itself, which is the exact opposite of what we are trying to achieve by stretching. If you bounce when you stretch, it can also mean that you stretch too deeply.

Rather than bouncing, you should try to elongate into your stretch. Hold the stretch for at least 20 seconds before releasing and then repeating. You might also want to practice dynamic stretching instead of bouncing.

Not Stretching Enough

Stretching is essential for everyone! The aim of stretching for you should be to maintain mobility and flexibility in your muscles and joints. If you don't stretch enough, then your muscles may shorten, and you could become limited in the movements you can do, feeling stiffer and in more discomfort as a result. If you include moderate amounts of stretching into your daily plan, this will help you move easier and reduce any chronic pain.

Holding Your Breath

You may not know this, but conscious breathing can result in a much more effective stretch. Often, people tend to unintentionally hold their breath when they are stretching, which, as a result, can lead to the muscles becoming resistant and tense. On the flip side, as you breathe, you are increasing your blood flow and providing your muscles with oxygen. By taking deep breaths slowly through your nose as you stretch, then your muscles will have more chance to relax and become more receptive to the stretch you are performing.

Stretching an Injured Muscle

Despite what you may have been told, stretching one of your injured muscles will not aid with reducing pain and can actually delay how long it will take for you to heal. Damaged tissue needs a break to make sure that it can heal.

Make sure to rest your injury, and instead look to use ice or heat as needed to help with your recovery. Once the injury has fully healed, that is when you can slowly add low intensity stretching of that muscle group back into the workout plan.

Chapter 8: Lifestyle and Philosophy

"Most persons are so absorbed in the contemplation of the outside world that they are wholly obvious to what is passing on within themselves." - Nikola Tesla

Why Everybody Needs a Life Philosophy

If you ever find yourself feeling overburdened by your share of daily activities, then this question could feel like it doesn't make sense.

You may think you have a lot of things that you are pursuing right now, a large series of goals, lots of commitments, a host of unfinished projects and deadlines. With all that on your plate, where is the fun in including philosophy to this already far too long list?

You might think that once you have got everything into a manageable place, you could already have the benefit of tackling a life philosophy then instead.

However, there are people out there that have no issue with answering this question confidently and with certainty. That is what we want. All aspects of your life will become clearer if you bring a new level of clarity to each of your goals.

It's not so much about what you get completed today, tomorrow, or even over the following year. It's more about what you are looking to get out of your life. What steps are you taking now that are going to help make this a reality?

If you aren't already taking those steps, then what is it that is stopping you from changing that?

Clarity

Having a clear, well-structured, and defined philosophy provides you with the boundaries and guidelines that you need to stay on track. It is important to have a specific philosophy, as it will help guide and drive each of your everyday actions.

You can view your philosophy as a lifelong commitment that will take you past simple self-improvement aspirations. The overall aim here is to achieve a radical transformation of yourself and, as a result, society.

All of this becomes possible once you allow yourself to explore the purpose and meaning of life in an attempt to find your place within the universe. Let's say, for example, that your philosophy is to execute things better than people have done previously. Imagine this is your top-tier goal, your guiding point that provides meaning and direction to each of the goals below it.

To achieve this top-tier goal, it may be required that you achieve many low-level and mid-level goals to get there. For example, a low-level goal may be making sure you leave the house by seven am. As a result, that will help you achieve a mid-level goal, in this instance, getting to work on time.

Why is that important? Because you would like to be punctual. Why do you care about being punctual? Because making sure you are punctual shows your respect for the other people that you work with. Why is it important to show respect? Because placed on your visionary board somewhere is a desire to become a good leader.

Having a clear philosophy lets you identify what it is you truly care about. When you are aware that you care about something, then you become loyal and consistent in pursuing that ultimate goal.

Every day, you will wake up thinking about the same series of questions that were in your head when you fell asleep the night before. You are consistently pointing in the same direction, always eager to try and take even the smallest step towards your goal.

One core belief that I always try to stick to that has served me well over the years is that you should focus all of your attention on the things that you have control over and accept that there are some things that are out of your control and that you can do nothing about.

This basic belief that I have practiced throughout my daily life has provided great increments in my efficacy whilst also reducing my levels of frustration.

Utility

When you find yourself in uncomfortable territory, you can feel as though things are not going towards your plan and you may feel constantly overwhelmed by a series of external events. Now more than ever, you need to dig deep and draw on the strength of your philosophy.

Say your worst fear is that you might lose your job. It can be tempting to play the victim, blaming things such as the economy, and fall into a never-ending cycle of complaining. Or you can accept that this is the reality and begin the search for what is next for you.

On the flip side, when you find yourself in your happy space, then this is the time that you need your philosophy to ensure that you stay on track.

Sanity

There is every possibility that some people may deem your focus to be obsessive, as almost all of your actions will be made with your life philosophy at the forefront of your mind. Obsessive is not the right wording; a better choice would be to say that you have got your priorities in order.

In people that are extremely committed, almost all of their low-level and mid-level goals relate to what their ultimate goal is. By contrast, those that have a lack of perseverance and commitment also tend to have a weaker coherent goal structure.

However, the concept that our entire life should be completely guided by a single top-level goal can be an idealized extreme and might not be what we want, even the craziest and the grittiest of us!

Still, I'd still say that it is more than possible to write down a lengthy list of low-level and mid-level work goals in accordance with how they serve your main goal. The more aligned, coordinated and unified your goal hierarchy is, the better.

But that doesn't mean that you shouldn't step back and pause every now and then for clarity of mind and your own sanity.

Pause for a moment and try to be in the present from time to time. I always tell people that you should try and appreciate each day as if you have just survived a car crash. A dramatic way of looking at it, but one that will help you have a greater appreciation for the little things in life.

And always make sure that you aren't putting your happiness on the back burner.

Benefits of Exercise in your Lifestyle

Everyone is looking for that miracle cure. The one that will reduce your chances of getting major illnesses like strokes, type 2 diabetes, heart disease, and cancer. A cure that can lower your chances of dying early.

We want something that will make an immediate impact, and without the hassle of meeting with a primary practice doctor. Unfortunately, there is only one thing that fits the bill and will help you with all of this, and that is exercise.

We can view exercise as the miracle cure that has always been available to us, but all too often, we neglect to do the amount that we should see these benefits. Regardless of how old you are, there is plenty of evidence to suggest that taking up physical exercise can play a major role in you living a happier and healthier life.

Not only that, but physical exercise is an excellent way to improve your mood, boost your self-esteem, increase your energy levels, and get a better night's sleep.

Health Benefits

On the whole, people who choose to exercise often have less of a chance of getting a lot of long-term issues, such as diabetes, stroke, heart disease, and some cancer.

Due to the overwhelming amount of evidence of the subject, it seems so clear that we should all try to be physically active. It is a key component if you are seeking to live a fulfilling and healthy life into old age.

On top of that, it can also reduce the risk of depression, stress, Alzheimer's disease, and dementia.

What Counts?

In order to keep healthy, you should try and be active as often as reasonably possible, completing at least three thirty-minute workouts each week using a variety of different methods.

For a lot of people, the simplest way to get more movement into your day to day life is to choose cycling or walking rather than a car to get around town.

However, the more you are able to do, the better, and doing more activities such as exercise and sport will allow you to become healthier.

To ensure you get the benefits from any activities you undertake, you need to make sure that you are moving fast enough to increase your heart rate, feel warmer, and breathe faster. This amount of effort is known as moderate-intensity activity. If you are working at this level, then you should be able to chat if needed, but you would struggle to sing along to a song.

An activity in which you are required to work harder than that is known as a vigorous-intensity activity. There is plenty of evidence to show that vigorous activity can lead to health benefits that are above and beyond what you can get from moderate activity. You will know when you are undertaking vigorous activity, as you will be breathing fast and hard, and your heart rate will have risen significantly. If you are working out at this level, then you will not be able to speak more than a couple of words without being forced to take a breath.

A Modern Problem

In general, people are not as active today as we once were. Technology has made life much easier, with most of us either driving cars or taking public transport rather than walking. We no longer wash our own clothes, as a machine does it for us, and we often entertain ourselves by sitting in front of a screen rather than being outside playing. Few people do manual work, and a lot of us have jobs that require little to no physical exertion.

Household chores, shopping, work, and many other vital activities are a lot less demanding than they were for previous generations.

As a result, we tend to move around less and therefore burn off fewer calories.

Sedentary Lifestyles

Inactivity is often referred to by experts as a silent killer. Living a sedentary life, such as lying or sitting down for large periods, is very bad for your health.

Inactivity is described by the Department of Health as a "silent killer". Evidence is emerging that sedentary behavior, such as sitting or lying down for long periods, is bad for your health.

That is why it is important to not only increase your activity levels but also try to decrease the time that you spend sitting down or lounging around.

Some of the most common examples of living a sedentary life include spending a lot of time on the computer, watching a lot of T.V., using the car instead of walking short journeys, and sitting down often to talk, read, or listen to music. This sedentary behavior is believed to increase the chances of developing a fair amount of chronic diseases, such as stroke, type 2 diabetes, and heart disease, as well as potentially suffering from unwanted weight gain.

Even if you hit your targeting amount of weekly activity, you could still be at risk of becoming ill or suffering from these issues if you spend all of your other time lying or sitting down.

Building your Lifestyle

The most difficult aspect of creating an exercise habit is actually to begin exercising. If you rely solely on motivation and willpower as a tactic, then you are doomed to fail before you even start.

Habits are actions that we take regardless of how motivated we feel or not. All too often, people seek out motivation boards and various exercise quotes to force themselves out to exercise. I've listed out some of the best habits that will stop you from depending on other people to begin exercising and continue living a life you enjoy.

Make your Goals Super Easy

As you begin your brand-new exercise journey, the first step you should take is to set some S.M.A.R.T. goals. These are goals that are smart, measurable, attainable, realistic, and timely. Ensure that these goals are extremely simple and easy so that you give yourself the best chance to get off to a good start.

You should treat these goals as your foundation, your building blocks. Seek to set goals that are as specific as they possibly can be. The more definitive that you make your goal, the more chance you have to succeed with that goal. For example, if you are desperate to run a marathon, yet you haven't gone out running in the last three months, then your first goal should be to run a mile at least twice a week.

Start Small and Build from There

It is much easier to implement lifestyle changes if you choose to take them one step at a time. There is absolutely no shame in starting with small goals, so long as you are meeting those goals and continue to progress them when the time comes. All too often, people fall into the trap of setting outrageously high ambitions with their habits, only to fall short and become demotivated.

It is better to become a master of a few habits rather than not mastering any at all. If you are brand new to working out and exercising, then make your new habit foolproof by committing to just thirty minutes, three times a week.

Thirty minutes does not seem like a large number, and the commitment level is low, which will lead to more chances of your succeeding, as these tasks are easy to begin with. Complete this goal of 30 minutes that will lead to more confidence in yourself, and before you know it, you will be doing 45 minutes and then an hour.

Log and Track your Habits

You can't class yourself as serious about achieving your goals until you begin tracking your progress. Making sure that you log your workouts is important as it is a way of showing you are going in the right direction or not and whether you need to make any adjustments.

How can you be sure that you are eating the right amount of food until you are keeping track of it? Tracking what you eat will allow you to adjust and manage your portions as required while also becoming more mindful of what you are putting into your body. Finally, take pictures and measurements on a monthly basis. This will add accountability to your training to remain on track. By choosing to take measurements and track your nutrition and workouts, then you create a great system of accountability, which in turn improves your chances of succeeding.

Find a Diet that is Easy, Sustainable, and Pleasing

There isn't a need to put yourself on a restrictive diet, where all of the food that you eat is boring and bland. To make sure that you are going to succeed with a healthier diet, then you should choose ways of eating that mix with your current lifestyle and not change it. Drastic diets can be harmful to the body, instead focus on making small changes such as drinking less alcohol in the week, not having dessert with an even meal as much, and other small changes.

Pick an Exercise Plan that Fits your Lifestyle

How often should you be working out a week? What training should you be doing? The answers to both of these questions will be dependent on your individual lifestyle. You don't need to spend every day in the gym; you can get great results from working out as little as three times a week, thirty minutes at a time. If you decide you only want to lift three days a week, then the push, pull, legs workout is ideal for that type of training plan. Remember, exercise should fit into your everyday life, not the other way around.

Find Fun Ways to Stay Active

Who said you need to hit the gym to be able to exercise? Whether you are cycling in the countryside, going hiking with friends, going out for a run, or even skipping out on getting in the elevator and instead of walking up the stairs, there are numerous ways to keep active and still burn calories.

Ways to Live a More Active Life

Making sure that your life is an active life is essential to maintain your health. As I have already noted, keeping yourself active will lower the chances of getting diabetes, heart disease, and stroke. Exercise has also been proved to increase your cognitive function and mental health.

You don't have to be a marathon runner to increase your health. It is important to ensure that you stay active, though. It will help you keep your strength, workout your heart, and keep a healthy weight.

The trick is to find a way of working out that you enjoy. For some people, that may be working out in the gym; for some, it could be walking around the block, and for others, it might be dancing around to an aerobics DVD in your living room; the main thing is just to get moving.

It can be hard to find your workout style. It can help to mix it up every once in a while. You may find that you like trying something new. Here are some simple strategies you can use to get active and stay active.

Take it Slow

If you haven't been very active in recent years, then it is important to start slowly. Make sure that you take all of the necessary precautions before you start exercising again. Overall, you will want to begin with short sessions that you can increase gradually over time as your body becomes more used to exercising again.

Get Your Thirty

Your aim for physical exercise should be 30 minutes, three times a week. This can be done in one 30-minute workout, or it could be done in two 15-minute sessions, or even three ten minute sessions.

Of course, exercising more than this is fine! But make sure you take all of the necessary precautions to prevent injuries, such as straining a muscle.

Work your Muscles

You shouldn't just be doing aerobic exercise. Weightlifting and resistance training is also an important part of any workout program. These types of training will help you increase your muscle and bone strength, as well as improving your coordination and balance. The lowers the chances of you getting osteoporosis and also reduces the chances of you getting injured.

Mix it up

A lot of community centers and gyms provide free gym classes as part of their monthly membership. You should take advantage of these free classes. You will likely experience new ways of training that you can implement into the rest of your workout plan to keep your motivation levels high.

You never know; you might become a fitness class fanatic as a result!

Mind your Money

You don't have to spend all your hard-earned cash to get a great workout in. If you aren't confident in going to a gym, fitness DVDs are an excellent way to workout, and a lot of local libraries stock copies that you will be able to rent. Check out different workout DVDs to give yourself an idea of what type of workouts you enjoy doing the most.

There are also plenty of fitness shows that are broadcast on T.V. or social media. Exercises classes come in all shapes and sizes, and all are available online for people, regardless of their fitness levels.

Stretch

Stretching at the end of a workout needs to be an essential part of your workout routine. As we have covered, stretching improves your range of motion and flexibility, and it can also reduce the chances of getting muscle cramps or getting injured. Finally, stretching also increases your blood circulation around the body.

The Takeaway

Keeping active is one of the essential aspects of maintaining a healthy lifestyle. As you get older, this becomes more and more important. Don't forget; you can get creative about how you fit in your exercise each day. You can dance around your lounge while you listen to the local news, you can choose to walk instead of drive to the grocery store, or take a quick walk after dinner.

Add in some strength training on the side to improve your muscle and bone strength, and you will be on your way to a better and healthier lifestyle.

Conclusion

And there you have it! Everything you could possibly need to know to make a positive change for good through exercise. You now have several different exercises that you can capitalize on to make yourself mentally and physically fitter. In each chapter, we have discussed many different exercises that you can do that will take your fitness levels to a new level.

We have also split these into different categories, for those of you that want to train from the comfort of your own home, or for those that have or want to get a gym membership, and have access to equipment such as barbells and cable machines.

For each chapter, there is a good variety of both home and gym workouts, which give you flexibility over your training. If you are a regular gym goer, but for whatever reason, you are struggling for time to drive to and from the gym, then there are plenty of exercises for each muscle group highlighted in this book for you to get an equally good workout at home.

Remember, I am not expecting or asking you to start training every single day. It is unreasonable to expect yourself to go from little to no training, to training every single day. It will severely impact the lifestyle that you are used to, and in the long run, it will demotivate you and probably leave you back to not training again, and we don't want that!

Not only that but overtraining and not allowing your muscles to recover can lead to overworking your muscles, which can leave you much more susceptible to injury. Getting injured will prevent you from training for longer periods of time, which can make it hard to restart again when you are fit as you may be all the way back at square one.

That is why it is also so important that you make sure you focus on keeping your form great throughout every single repetition of every single movement. Even when you have done an exercise multiple times, do not become complacent with your form, as this is what will help prevent you from getting injured, and also ensure that you are working the right muscle groups for what you are trying to achieve.

This becomes especially important as you increase the amount of weight that you have on the bar. The heavier the weight, the more important your form becomes because the more pressure you will be putting on your body. Keeping good for should always be at the top of your priority list. Park your ego at the door and accept that some people might lift bigger weights than you. Trust in the process and you will be lifting those weights in no time, and if they are using the incorrect form to lift that weight then they either won't be getting the benefits or will find themselves injured very soon.

Another absolutely vital aspect of any lifestyle that is looking to implement a healthy exercise plan, is to make sure that you have a solid set of habits in place. Good habits are required to make sure that you stay on track and keep to your new exercise goals. Without good habits in place, it can be all too easy to fall off your plan, and as soon as you do that it can be really difficult to get everything back on track.

Good habits to take on board are to take things slow, don't set out goals that you aren't going to be able to achieve really easily at first. It might seem counterproductive to set really low goals, as you are likely extremely keen and motivated right now. But we need to set goals that you can achieve even when life gets in the way or your motivation simply isn't there. That way, you will stay on track and stay positive with your training.

If you set workout plans that are difficult to maintain week in week out, then ultimately you will start to miss your targets. If you miss your targets, even if you are still doing a lot of exercise, you will find that you become demotivated as you feel that you are failing. That feeling of failure that you begin to associate with exercising is more than likely going to lead to you giving up on your workout plan sooner than you should have.

A more long term sustainable approach is to start slowly and build up your workout volume as you become more confident with your plan week in week out.

Another good habit you should get into is making sure that you mix up your workouts. By making sure that you don't do the same workouts more than a couple of times in a row, you will make sure that workouts stay fun and interesting, and you won't become bored of doing the same thing, over and over again. By doing the same workouts day in, day out, you are setting yourself up to get bored much quicker with exercising, making yourself more likely to give up.

Not only that but working the same muscles each workout will allow your body to adapt to the exercises. This will lead to you gaining less and less benefit from each training session. If you aren't seeing the same results then that can also lead to you becoming demotivated.

Making sure that you mix up your workouts is essential to keep your body on its toes, and continue to make progress in your workout program. These are just some of the reasons that it is essential to set up good habits to stay on track with your exercise goals.

As we have discussed, motivation is so important for anything you do in life, and this is no different from exercise. If you are not motivated to train, it can be much harder to bring yourself to do your workout for the day. And if you don't complete the workout for that day, that can lead to further demotivation down the line, as you feel as though you aren't hitting your targets.

Remember, anything that you do, even if it's a 15-minute walk, is better than what you were doing previously, which was likely nothing. Don't compare what you have achieved in a day to what you might have achieved. Instead, compare it to whether you had done nothing. Keep this perspective at the forefront of your mind, and you will stay motivated to keep working on your goals.

It is also always handy to remind yourself from time to time what the reason was that made you want to start exercising. Was it to lose a little extra weight? Was it to lower your chances of disease? The truth is it doesn't matter what your goal is as that is personal to you. What does matter is making sure that you remind yourself of your "why" from time to time, as this will keep you motivated.

Finally, think about the topic we covered in our final chapter of this book, ensuring that you have a life philosophy in place. Life philosophies are essential as they give your life meaning and purpose, and something that you can strive towards each and every day, and with everything that you do.

Each decision that you make can be based around ultimately achieving this goal, and having it in place will give you clarity on what you should and shouldn't be doing to try and achieve it.

Is the action or task going to take you a step closer to your life goal? If not that you should seriously consider whether it is worth doing or not. This will bring clarity to your life where you need it most.

And that's everything! I hope you enjoyed reading my book, and you are able to start actioning all of the things that you have learned, and change your life for the better, through daily exercise.

References

Barroso, M. (2017, January 25). 8 Exercises for Incredible Grip Strength. Medium. https://medium.com/@Mark_Barroso/8-exercises-for-incredible-grip-strength-a44d05bca432

Bedosky, L. (2019, October 29). Chest Anatomy: What Are The Muscles And What Do They Do. Openfit. https://www.openfit.com/chest-muscles

Bill Geiger. (2016, July 30). 10 Best Chest Exercises For Building Muscle | Bodybuilding.com. Bodybuilding.com; Bodybuilding.com. https://www.bodybuilding.com/content/10-best-chest-exercises-for-building-muscle.html

Bubnis, D. (2020, June 2). 21 At-Home Bicep Exercises for Captain America Arms. Greatist. https://greatist.com/health/bicep-workouts-at-home#bodyweight-and-resistance-bands

Carrier, K. (2018, July 18). The Biggest Mistakes You're Making During Leg Workouts. Www.Jerseystrong.com. https://www.jerseystrong.com/blog/biggest-mistakes-youre-making-during-leg-workouts

Harrison, L. (2016, June 16). 7 Exercises to Maximize Hand, Wrist, and Forearm Strength. Breaking

Muscle. https://breakingmuscle.com/fitness/7-exercises-to-maximize-hand-wrist-and-forearm-strength

Hobbs, W. (2018, July 12). Leg Muscles Anatomy, Function & Diagram | Body Maps. Healthline. https://www.healthline.com/human-body-maps/leg-muscles#2

Jacobs, M. (2017, December 24). Muscles of the Pectoral Region. TeachMeAnatomy. https://teachmeanatomy.info/upper-limb/muscles/pectoral-region/

Mateo, A. (2019, April 10). The Best At-Home Exercises for a Stronger Back | Everyday Health. EverydayHealth.com. https://www.everydayhealth.com/fitness/best-home-exercises-stronger-back/#:~:text=Push%20your%20hips%20back%2C%20knees

Mobin, A. (2018, November 28). Bicep Training: The Top 5 Mistakes to Avoid. AS-IT-IS Nutrition. https://asitisnutrition.com/blogs/health/bicep-training-the-top-5-mistakes-to-avoid

Parker Hyde. (2016, July 17). 10 Best Muscle-Building Back Exercises! | Bodybuilding.com. Bodybuilding.com; Bodybuilding.com. https://www.bodybuilding.com/content/10-best-muscle-building-back-exercises.html

Root, T. (2018, September 20). Shoulder Muscles Anatomy, Diagram & Function | Body Maps. Healthline. https://www.healthline.com/human-body-maps/shoulder-muscles#2

Rothschild, M. (2014, April 8). 5 Common Cardiovascular Training Mistakes to Avoid. Rock Creek Sports Club. https://rockcreeksportsclub.com/5-common-cardiovascular-training-mistakes-to-avoid/

Sawyers, J. (2019, April 10). The Muscles of the Hand - Thenar - Hypothenar - TeachMeAnatomy. Teachmeanatomy.Info. https://teachmeanatomy.info/upper-limb/muscles/hand/

Smith, P. (2017, August 30). 10 Best Shoulder Exercises for Your Home Workout. Openfit. https://www.openfit.com/shoulder-workouts-at-home

Stanley, J. (2020, July 7). 7 Exercises to Avoid in Your Legs Workouts. Muscle & Fitness. https://www.muscleandfitness.com/workouts/leg-exercises/7-moves-avoid-your-leg-workouts/

Stevens, D. (2018, July 31). Preventing Injury: 8 Best Hand and Wrist Exercises for Computer Users. Ergonomic Trends. http://ergonomictrends.com/hand-wrist-exercises-computer-users/

Stilwell, B. (2020, June 24). 5 of the best shoulder exercises you should be doing in the gym. We Are The Mighty. https://www.wearethemighty.com/mighty-fit/5-of-the-best-shoulder-exercises-you-should-be-doing-in-the-gym/?rebelltitem=1#rebelltitem1

Washmuth, D. (2019, March 2). Triceps Brachii Muscle: Definition, Function & Location | Study.com. Study.com. https://study.com/academy/lesson/triceps-brachii-muscle-definition-function-location.html

Webb, D. (2018, January 4). 30 Best Leg Exercises and Leg Workouts of All Time. Men's Journal. https://www.mensjournal.com/health-fitness/30-best-leg-exercises-and-workouts-of-all-time/5-dumbbell-stepup/

Whyle, J. (2014, February 8). The Superficial Back Muscles - Attachments - Actions - TeachMeAnatomy. Teachmeanatomy.Info. https://teachmeanatomy.info/back/muscles/superficial/

Wood, M. (2018, September 14). Triceps Anatomy, Origin & Function | Body Maps. Healthline. https://www.healthline.com/human-body-maps/triceps#1

Woodhead, J. (2017, July 22). Chest Workout: At Home With and Without Equipment. 8fit.

https://8fit.com/fitness/chest-workout-at-home-with-without-equipment/

Yeung, A. (2018, April 5). 10 Bench-Press Mistakes Killing Your Progress. Muscle & Fitness. https://www.muscleandfitness.com/workouts/workout-tips/10-bench-press-mistakes-are-killing-your-progress/

www.ingramcontent.com/pod-product-compliance
Lightning Source LLC
Chambersburg PA
CBHW032134020426
42334CB00016B/1162